AMANI
Birth

Assisting Mothers for Active, Natural, Instinctive Birth

BY

AISHA AL HAJJAR

AMANI
Birth

Assisting Mothers for Active, Natural, Instinctive Birth

DEDICATION

It is with all praises to *Allah* (*SWT*) that this work is dedicated for His sake to all Muslim Mothers, Fathers, and their children, whether born or unborn. This is a sister-to-sister, mother-to-mother resource and I pray that *Allah* provides the best of it and protects from any harm in it. May your births be easy and your children healthy and pleasing to Him and their parents... *Ameen*!

TABLE OF CONTENTS

Dedication	v
Disclaimer	xi
Important Islamic Teachings	xii
Islamic Vocabulary	xiii
Acknowledgements	xvii
Books Available	xx
Bio and Vision	xxi
My Personal Journey	xxv
What is AMANI?	1
Part One - Assisting	3
Chapter 1 – History of Medical Birth Attendants	5
Chapter 2 – AMANI Birth Attendants	9
Chapter 3 – Childbirth Education	15
Chapter 4 – Family and Friends as Labor Companions	25
Chapter 5 – Professional Labor Companions	37
Chapter 6 – What to Expect in AMANI Birth Training-Part One	43
Part Two - Mothers	49
Chapter 7 – Who is AMANI Birth for?	51

Chapter 8 – Physiology of Pregnancy   53

Chapter 9 – Physiology of Labor and Birth   61

Chapter 10 – Enjoying the Birth Experience   71

Chapter 11 – Postpartum Recovery   75

Chapter 12 – The Baby's Needs and Rights   91

Chapter 13- What to Expect in AMANI Birth Training-Part Two   97

Part Three - Active   99

Chapter 14 – Pregnancy Nutrition and Exercise   101

Chapter 15 – Birth Consumerism   115

Chapter 16 – Freedom of Movement and Birth Positions   121

Chapter 17 – Minimizing and Coping With Pain   131

Chapter 18 - What to Expect in AMANI Birth Training-Part Three   137

Part Four - Natural   141

Chapter 19 – Labor Has a Purpose   143

Chapter 20 – Birth is Inherently Safe   147

Chapter 21 – Birth is Not without Risk   151

Chapter 22 – Birth is Not without Pain   161

Chapter 23 – Dangers of Interventions   175

Chapter 24 – Points to Minimize Interventions   199

Chapter 25 - What to Expect in AMANI Birth Training-Part Four   203

Part Five – Instinctive   205

Chapter 26 – Hawwaa and Maryam (Eve and Mary)   207

Chapter 27 – Emotions, Environment, and Hormones   209

Chapter 28 – Follow Your Instincts, Trust Allah   215

Chapter 29 – Breastfeeding and Baby Care   219

Chapter 30 – What to Expect in AMANI Birth Training-Part Five   245

References: 249

Disclaimer

It's important to note that this is not intended to be a medical reference or to replace professional care during pregnancy, labor, or birth. The purpose is to explore the natural and normal functions of birth with trust in the design of the female body to carry out this function. Each woman should consider her personal situation and medical history and work closely with her birth team to achieve the safest and best birth experience for her and her baby, wherever and with whomever it takes place.

Allah (*SWT*) has given us bodies to birth and medical interventions for the <u>rare</u> complications that may arise. We pray that this book will be a source of confidence and encouragement to employ those interventions only when <u>truly</u> necessary.

We cannot stress enough the importance of good birth consumerism by women who are educated and empowered to keep control of the decisions of their birth and make the best decisions for their particular situations. You have choices in birth; not making any choice is a choice that allows someone else full control over your experience and outcome.

I am also not an Islamic scholar and there is no intended or implied *fatwa* (ruling or opinion) in this material. Feedback and references are welcomed for revised editions.

Tie your camel and put your trust in *Allah*: get educated and choose wisely and cautiously. Your baby, your recovery, your family, and our worldwide community depend on it!

Important Islamic Teachings

One day Prophet Muhammad (sallallaahu 'alayhi wa sallam) noticed a Bedouin leaving his camel without tying it and he asked the Bedouin, "Why don't you tie down your camel?" The Bedouin answered, "I put my trust in Allah." The Prophet then said, "Tie your camel first, then put your trust in Allah." [At-Tirmidhi]

"...Verily never will Allah change the condition of a people until they change it themselves..." [Qur'an 13:11]

This *hadith* (saying of the Prophet Muhammad, **sallallaahu 'alayhi wa sallam**) and *ayah* (verse) teach us to prepare as much as we can and then trust the will of *Allah (SWT)*. It is important that we do our part in preparation for birth, just as for all areas of our lives.

Islamic Vocabulary

Alayhas-Salam/ Alayhis-Salām: Peace upon her/him

Alhamdulillah: Thanks to Allah

Allah: God

Allahu Akbar: Allah is the Most Great

Allahu A'lam: Allah knows

AMANI: Wishes

AMANI *lil Banaat*: Wishes for Girls

AMANI *lil Welada Tabiaya*: Wishes for Natural Birth

Ameen: Amen

astaghfirullah: May Allah forgive me!

Athan/adhan: Call for prayer

A'uthubillah: I seek protection

Ayat/Ayah: The verses of the Quran, but it can also mean proofs, evidences, lessons, signs, revelations, miracles, etc.

Bedouin: An Arab of any of the nomadic tribes of the Arabian, Syrian, Nubian, or Sahara Deserts

Bismillah: In the name of Allah

Bukhari, Muslim, Sahih Bukhari, Sahih Muslim, Musnad Ahmad At-Tirmidhi, Ibn Majah Ahmad, Nasai: Books of authentic Prophetic narrations

fardh: Obligatory

Fatwa: A religious verdict

fiqh: Islamic jurisprudence

Ghusl: Ritual bath

Hadith/hadeeth: Narrations of the Prophet

halal: Permitted in Islam

Hanafi, Maliki, Shafi'and Hanbali: School of thoughts of Islamic law

haram: Forbidden in Islam

hasanat/hasanah: Rewards

in sha' Allah: With Allah's Will

iqamah: Second call to start the prayer

Islam: The true way of worshiping God, literally means peace, purity, submission, and obedience

istikharah: A prayer to ask for Allah's guidance

Jinn: supernatural spirits mentioned in the Quran who inhabit an unseen world in dimensions beyond the visible universe of humans. They are made of a smokeless and "scorching fire," and they have the physical property of weight. Like human beings, the jinn can also be good, evil, or neutrally benevolent.

Jumu'ah: Friday, but may also refer to the Friday prayer.

Ka'bah: The Holy Sanctuary in Makkah

Magian: A member of the Zoroastrian priestly caste of the Medes and Persians

masjid: Mosque

ma sha' Allah: With Allah's Grace

Makkah: The holy city

Tuhfat al-Mawdud bi Ahkam al-Mawlud: Name of an Islamic book

Qur'an: Allah's revelations to the Prophet

Radiallahu Anhu: May Allah be pleased with him

"All-ahumma aslamtu nafsi ilaika, wa wajjahtu wajhi ilaika, wa fauwadtu Amri ilaika, wa alja'tu zahri ilaika, raghbatan warahbatan ilaika. La Malja'a wa la manja minka illa ilaika. Amantu bikitabika al-ladhi anzalta wa nabi-yyika al-ladhi arsalta!

A Prayer that means: O Allah! I surrender to You and entrust all my affairs to You and depend upon You for Your Blessings both with hope and fear of You. There is no fleeing from You, and there is no place of protection and safety except with You O Allah! I believe in Your Book (the Qur'an) which You have revealed and in Your Prophet (Muhammad) whom You have sent.

Acknowledgements

All praises and thanks are to *Allah* (*SWT*). It is with full acknowledgment of Him that this work is submitted and I pray it is accepted and beneficial for all who read it. Anything good in this work is from Him and any error is my own.

Acknowledgments are due to Jay and Marjie Hathaway, cofounders of the American Academy of Husband-Coached Childbirth® (AAHCC). Through their lifework, I learned what I needed to tie my camels and enjoy the eight beautiful births I've been blessed by *Allah* (*SWT*) to experience. They also served as my first teachers in the realm of natural birth professionalism and I cannot thank them enough! Additionally, acknowledgement is due to the late Dr. Bradley, upon whose work the AAHCC® is based. I also hold special appreciation for Janet Carrol, my personal Bradley Method® teacher during my first pregnancy.

Sincere gratitude is due to Dr. Sarah Buckley of Australia for her support of natural birth. Her work has been pivotal in my growth and her kindness and generosity are greatly appreciated!

Sincere appreciation is also afforded to Janet Balaskas, author of *Active Birth*. Her writing enlightened me to think beyond the work of Dr. Bradley and the AAHCC®. I am also encouraged by her personal achievements in affecting change in the birthing culture of her community. She is truly an inspiration! Likewise, enough cannot be said about the inspirational writings and work of Ina May Gaskin, Jan Tritten, Dr. Marsden Wagner, and Ricki Lake. All four are a resonating voice for the midwifery model of care and support of a woman's right to birth naturally. Gratitude is also extended to the numerous contributors to Midwifery Today magazine and speakers at their international conferences, where I have learned so much.

In addition to Dr. Bradley, Dr. Buckley, and Dr. Wagner, I would like to thank the many doctors who are gems amongst the rocks, who have kept my faith in the medical professional's ability to support natural birth. To name just a few, the late Dr. Thomas Brewer of the United States, Dr. Fernando Molina, of Venezuela, Dr. Hanna Abo Kassem of Egypt, and Dr. Michel Odent of France. I am sure there are many more out there and I would love to be in touch.

I cannot say enough about the fabulous growth and exposure that I have experienced through my writing opportunities on Saudi Life. In fact, extra special appreciation is due to Akhy Faraz, Dr. Rahla, Umm Zakiyyah, Ukhty Afifa and the rest of the Saudi Life family for all their support and encouragement. May Allah continue to bless Saudi Life and may it be of great benefit to the *Ummah* (*Muslim* community).

Personal thanks are due to the circle of Doulas, Breastfeeding Counselors, and other birth professionals I have met and worked with in Saudi Arabia. Annelyse, Ihsan, Hind, Lynette, Salma Umm Layla, Stacey, Alaa, Alicia, Dayle, Selma, Sarah, Andrea, Umm Badr, Umm Layth, Hodane, Makkah, Dr. Hessa, Anne, and Dr. Modia, you have all been a source of inspiration and your feedback and sisterly support has been monumental in this journey!

I am also eternally grateful to the fabulous staff and faculty at Midwives College of Utah where my journey to midwifery takes place. Kim, Nicole, Dianne, Kristi, Paula, Julie, Erin, Marilyn, April, Heather, Jes, Sonia, Cindy, Crystal, Chris, Felicia, Gayelynn, Danielle, Kaylee, and the others behind the scenes, thank you for your support and encouragement as you have worked hard to train me for the noble task of caring for women during their childbearing years. Additional acknowledgments are due to my sister midwifery students, especially Eudine, Regina, Angie, Sherry, Terah, Jessica, and too many more to mention, but who have cheered me on and encouraged me along my path and supported my studies and efforts. It is an honor and a privilege to share the path to midwifery at MCU. As well as to Sandi Blankenship, who served as one of my first clinical teachers of midwifery. Special thanks is due to Brenda, Budi, Gyna and the other midwives at Rumah Sehat Madani in Bali for their gracious support of my clinical studies in midwifery.

Heartfelt appreciation is everlasting to my supportive husband, Mohammed, without whom I would not have had the fortitude to finish this project. Likewise, my mother, who has been an unwavering support of my work and an instrumental help with my children. Special appreciation and endearment is due to my children, especially the older five who help me so much. Khalid, Sarah, Amina, Salman, Rayan, Haider, Faris, and this book's namesake, Amani, each of your births have been special just as each of you are to me. I have learned through the privilege of being your mother and pray our lessons can be of benefit to others.

BOOKS AVAILABLE

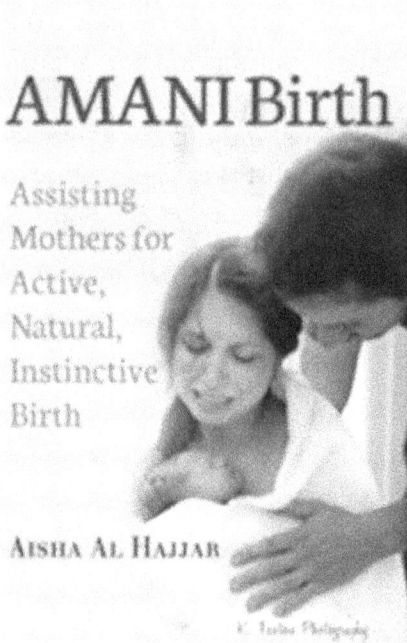

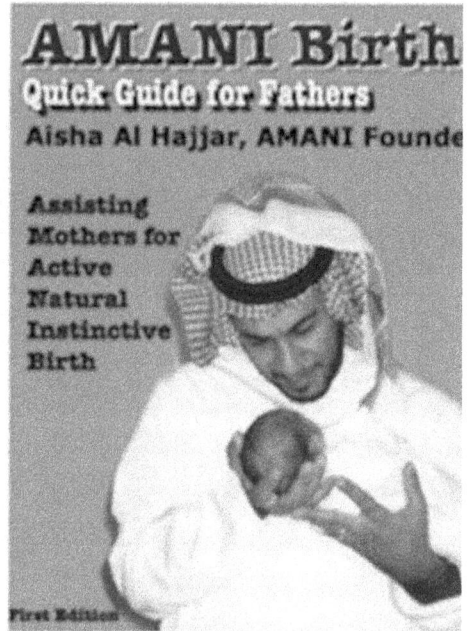

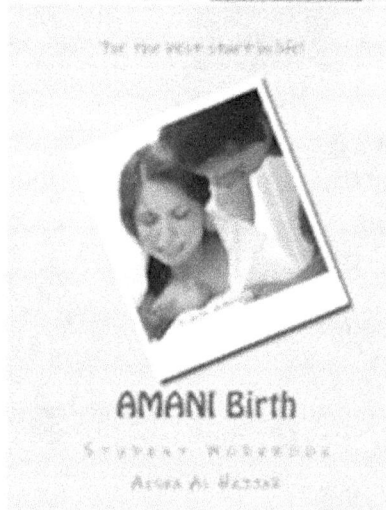

The workbook is only available from Certified AMANI Birth
Teachers for use in AMANI Childbirth classes.
Visit http://www.amanibirth.com for a teacher near you.

Bio and Vision

Aisha Al Hajjar is an American mother of eight beautiful children. She is married to Mohammed Al Hajjar from Saudi Arabia. Mohammed has grown to be the rock of support she needs to face the Middle Eastern birthing culture. Aisha and Mohammed currently reside in Riyadh, Saudi Arabia and put their trust in *Allah* (*SWT*) and ask HIS blessing of this work. May the *Muslim Ummah* (community) get the best from it and be protected from any harm...*AMEEN*.

Aisha discovered the passionate world of natural birthing through a distant acquaintance at the age of seventeen. At twenty-six, she birthed her first baby naturally, using the Bradley Method® of Natural Childbirth without pain medications, medical interventions, or episiotomy in a Sacramento, California hospital. A year and a half later, she discovered the power of her Bradley® training during her second birth in a Clovis, California hospital.

She went on to have three more children naturally in various hospitals in California before converting to *Islam* and moving to Alexandria, Egypt. There she birthed her sixth baby naturally amidst a very disturbing birthing culture. She had her seventh baby in Jeddah, Saudi Arabia. It was apparent that she was "allowed" to birth naturally only because she was American and she immediately felt her calling to bring natural childbirth education and advocacy to the Middle East.

During her eighth pregnancy she returned to America to train and certify as a Bradley Method® Teacher, Lecturer, and Professional Labor/Birth Companion (Doula). This set the foundation for her work in Egypt and Saudi Arabia. She has gone on to train as a Breastfeeding Counselor through the World Health Organization (WHO) and UNICEF program at the *Al Bidayah* Center in Saudi Arabia and is a founding member of Circle of Nurturing, a Mother-to-Mother *Islamic* Breastfeeding Support Group based in Riyadh, Saudi Arabia. At the time of this writing, she is also a midwifery student at Midwives College of Utah. She is finishing her academic study to earn a Bachelors of Science in Midwifery and completing the clinical portion of her study as a Midwife's Apprentice to various midwives at King Fahad Medical City Women's Specialized Hospital in Saudi Arabia. At the completion of her degree she anticipates also being registered with the North American Registry of Midwives (NARM) as a Certified Professional Midwife. She has also served as Midwife's Apprentice to Sandi Blankenship, Water Birth Guru, in Guangzhou, China, and as an Obstetrician's Midwife Assistant to Dr. Hanna Abo Kassem in Alexandria, Egypt.

Aisha became a voice for natural birth through her personal blog, Saudi Birth Story, and her Motherhood column on Saudi Life. She also has a Parenting column on Saudi Life and writes freelance features for Arab News. She has been blessed with these public forums where she shares her thoughts on birthing and provides a platform for other Muslim sisters to share their birth stories. She has kept herself available to the public and is happy to answer questions and provide natural childbirth education and doula services to anyone interested. She trains women to teach the AMANI Birth curriculum and to serve as AMANI Birth Doulas

Through her exploration, experiences, studies, and discoveries she set out to change the birthing culture of the Muslim *Ummah*. She initiated the AMANI Birth project to bring awareness and education to her Muslim sisters and brothers about the miracle of birth as *Allah* (SWT) has created it in HIS most infinite wisdom. It is her dream to bring AMANI Birth training to every Muslim family worldwide and to provide alternatives to hospital birthing with a string of quality natural birthing centers in the Middle East, starting in Saudi Arabia, *in sha' Allah*.

At the time of this writing, Aisha and her husband, Mohammed, are in the planning stages of opening AMANI Birth and Women's Wellness Community Center. Their vision is to function as a training center for AMANI Birth Professional Childbirth Educators/Doulas as well as provide AMANI Birth Childbirth Education to expectant parents. Another facet of the AMANI vision is the AMANI Girls Health, Nutrition, and Exercise programs that are geared towards preteen and teen girls to teach them the importance of good health during adolescence as a preparation for future motherhood and aging. Once Aisha graduates her midwifery program, the

Center will expand to provide well-women care from first menses to menopause, including pre- and post- natal care, and eventually grow into the first AMANI Low Risk Birth Center for out-of-hospital birthing, *in sha' Allah.*

Most importantly, Aisha believes that birth is a glorious act of worship and trust in the Creator and HIS perfect design of the female body to carry, birth, and feed our young. It is with all glory and gratitude to *Allah* (*SWT*) that this work is presented. *Alhamdulillah, subhan'Allah, Allahu Akbar!*

My Personal Journey

Before it all began...

My journey to help Muslim women have better birth experiences began long before the birth of my first son. I was about seventeen when I had the fortune to meet a woman who had four children. At the time that seemed like soooooooooo many! Of course, I could not foresee my own destiny to have eight (so far), *subhan'Allah*. Even more unforeseen was my future conversion to *Islam* and relocation halfway around the world to Saudi Arabia. If I had read my own story back then, I never would have recognized the writer as myself!

Looking back, I think what struck me about this mom-of-four was her passion around pregnancy and birth. During a brief conversation, she mentioned that her young daughter wanted to be a midwife. I was shocked that such a young child would even know what a midwife was, let alone aspire for such an unusual profession. When I asked her about this she told me that her older children had witnessed the births of the younger as she had delivered them all at home with a midwife. She also mentioned that she was training to be a Bradley Method® Childbirth Educator. Another vivid memory is of her rushing out of a social event all-aflutter about assisting a woman in labor with a homebirth, breech delivery.

At the time, I didn't understand much about her passions. I wasn't too keen about the whole homebirth idea, I mean after-all, everyone *knows* they are unsafe (or are they?). Home birth seemed so extreme amidst our current world of hospital and obstetrician centered birthing.

Even though I saw her as eccentric, I was drawn by her passionate approach to birth. It was unlike anyone else I knew. She seemed to love birth, while all the expectant moms I had ever known or seen in the media portrayed birth as a *terrifying event looming in their future.*

I didn't necessarily see myself as radical as she. "I mean, homebirth? Come on, that's just too much!" I thought. But I did know that someday, when my own turn came, I wanted the enthusiasm, passion, and excitement that she had.

Expecting my first...

I was twenty-five before I found myself expecting. I was thrilled and terrified all at the same time. I had always wanted children and had begun to wonder if I ever would. (Ha...look at me now, with eight, *alhamdulillah*!) I had mentally held on to the one thing that I had heard from my earlier experience that I hoped would link me to a better birth...*The Bradley Method*.

I had moved to another state by now and was hoping I could find out more from someone near me. Luckily, I found The Bradley Method's toll-free number listed in the phone directory. I called and was promised a teacher directory by post (pre-internet days, if you can imagine that!).

Janet Carrol was fresh out of training and teaching her first class. That didn't matter to me. I was just thrilled to find a teacher nearby. I had no idea what to expect or what I'd learn; I just knew that I didn't want to experience birth as a traumatic event like most all women had seemed to do before me. I knew from my earlier encounter that there must be a better way.

My husband and I faithfully attended classes, week after week. We learned exercises to prepare my body for the birth, nutrition to keep me healthy and low-risk, the physiology of pregnancy and birth, the dangers and misinformation given about drugs and medicinal pain relief, and most importantly how to work with my body to reduce pain and have the best all-natural, non-medicated birth experience possible.

I am eternally grateful that *Allah (SWT)* led me down this birthing path. I am fairly confident that had these seemingly random events (meeting the passionate birth mama when I was seventeen and taking classes when I became pregnant) not occurred, I would not have had the knowledge to prepare myself physically, emotionally, and mentally for my first birth experience. I truly believe without this knowledge, I would have suffered through my birth as most women do and not been so keen to repeat it!

After the birth of my son I felt great, a little sore, like bruising, but nothing I needed pain medication for. In fact, the doctor prescribed something and when the nurse brought it in I told her, "I just birthed without pain meds; you think I need it now?" She left it on my bedside table *just in case*. Of course, looking back I realize that this is one more money-making event that takes place as I'm sure my insurance company was charged a pretty-penny for those unused drugs!

Birthing my second...

About a year and a half later, I was back in the hospital to deliver my second baby. I had not given childbirth classes a second thought. After all, I did it all-natural last time so I know I can do it again. Right?!?

When I was in the midst of that second labor, I panicked. This was way harder than last time! It hurt so much more. My husband saw I was losing control and calmly said, "Remember to tummy breathe." That was all I needed. Upon hearing his words the whole gamut of Bradley® training came flooding back. I immediately responded with the techniques we had been taught and I realized a fifty percent reduction in my pain.

Right then and there, in the middle of a contraction, I thought, "Wow! I have control over just how much this hurts! There really is something to this stuff they teach!"

I gave some thought to becoming a Bradley® teacher myself, but the investment in time and money was just too much at that time of my life. Even so, it was an aspiration that I carried quietly inside as I went on to give birth naturally to babies three, four, and five.

My First Birth with my Saudi Husband...

Shortly after the birth of our fifth child, my marriage fell apart. The children and I suffered a lot of emotional terror and abuse from their father. It was during this time that I began seeking God. *Alhamdulillah*, after a year or so in dedication to Christianity, I found *Islam*.

As a divorcee with five children, I didn't expect to have any more babies. But Allah is the best of planners, *subhan'Allah*. I found myself living in Egypt, married to a Saudi, and expecting my sixth child. I was afraid of the care I might receive in the Egyptian hospitals and began looking for a midwife to deliver at home. I was surprised that I couldn't find anyone.

I decided to look up Bradley® on the Internet. I figured if there was a teacher there, surely she'd know of a good midwife in the area. I was sadly disappointed to find that there were no teachers anywhere near the region.

As I learned more about the birthing culture in Egypt, I began to seriously consider becoming a teacher. To top it off, I was devastated when my new husband announced, "In my culture, birth is a woman thing. I hope you don't mind, but I don't want to be with you when you deliver."

I was devastated. I couldn't believe he didn't want to be there for the birth of his child! What's more, I knew this was a time I would need him most. Especially since I was in a land and culture foreign to me and he knew I couldn't speak the language. I had no one else and I felt terribly abandoned.

Although I hated it, I birthed without him. I was fortunate to find a doctor who trusted my experience and allowed me to birth completely naturally, without pain medication or medical interference. I can't say enough about how much I love Dr. Mona for her respect and not trying to control my birth, *alhamdulillah*. However, I wasn't impressed with the birthing facility and especially the delivery table. I found myself in the most awkward and difficult position I had ever endured for birth. But it was birthing without my husband that really hurt. I must admit, it was the most emotionally painful birth I had experienced. Although it was also affirming to know that I could birth naturally, with or without the support of my husband.

Physically speaking, although the position was hard, I managed to get through it just fine, *alhamdulillah*. In fact, when I called to tell my husband that I had delivered and was home just two hours later making lunch for the kids, he felt bad. He was in Saudi and I was alone with five young children and a newborn. He really thought that I must be suffering and even confided in his closest coworker just how horrible he felt, knowing I had no one to help me.

Of course, he didn't realize that I really did feel physically fine, as he'd never known a woman who birthed truly naturally. His only experience was of women who were run over by medical interventions and pain medications and who truly could not care for themselves, let alone the new baby and other children, without several weeks of help. In fact, in Saudi culture, it's common for the woman to spend a few days in the hospital (if not longer) and then go to her mother's home where she is pampered and cared for during the first forty postpartum days. The husband is usually out of the picture during this time and only stops by to visit his recovering wife and new baby every few days. He simply couldn't believe I was home and functioning all alone within two hours of birth.

Determined to Home Birth...

With the seventh pregnancy I did not want to endure another horrible delivery table and I was now in Saudi, where I was skeptical that I'd find a doctor who'd be as receptive to my way of birthing as Dr. Mona had been. I was now emotionally prepared to birth alone. So much so, that I decided to do it completely alone at home. Thankfully, my husband supported my desire to birth at home. "So long as I don't have to participate," he conditionally agreed.

I was past the point of expecting his involvement. I just wanted to have my baby alone, and in peace. The thing that worried us both was getting the baby documented afterwards. My husband visited the various government Ministries to find out what would be needed to obtain a birth certificate. At each counter, he was met with shock and warnings of the "dangers" and how cumbersome the paperwork process would be. No one said it was illegal but it was obviously frowned upon.

Realizing that getting the baby documented would be difficult without a hospital record; we decided to visit a doctor to ask if she would attest to my pregnancy so that there would be no question of having given birth to my baby. As it turned out, I was unknowingly in active labor when I arrived for my appointment (I had been having false labor contractions for weeks with this pregnancy and did not recognize it as true labor). When the doctor announced that my husband should register me for the birth right then and there, I panicked. I was struggling to get up and calling his name. But he was long gone down the hall towards the admissions desk.

Just as I was trying to dress, my water broke and I felt my baby noticeably descend. I knew then that I wasn't going home until this was over. The staff quickly rushed a gurney to my bedside and coaxed me to slide onto it. They threw a heavy blanket over my body and head to guard my modesty and ran off, crashing into walls, towards the delivery room.

I ended up delivering during the wild ride on the rolling table. So in the end, Allah is the best of planners and it didn't work out for me to have a home-birth, *subhan'Allah*. But I did get to birth completely naturally, as there was no time for anyone to interfere. At the same time, since it happened in the hospital I was able to get the baby documented with ease, *alhamdulillah*.

The Birth of AMANI...

Just before I discovered my eighth pregnancy, I decided to pursue the calling to teach Bradley® classes in the Middle East. I submitted my application and booked our tickets for the trip to the States. Soon after my application was accepted, I realized I was expecting again, *alhamdulillah*.

My husband was incredibly supportive and listened as I read portions of my academic study out loud to him. Even more, I was pleasantly surprised when he agreed to meet with Janet, my Bradley® teacher of fifteen years back. She had offered us a rush refresher of the material before attending the teacher-training workshop in California. I was thrilled that he agreed and prayed he might learn something from the experience.

When it was time to attend the teacher's workshop my husband was faced with a dilemma: attend classes with me, or sit in the hotel room with seven children for several hours each day. Since there was one other husband sitting in with his wife, my husband decided to try it out. He wouldn't commit to the whole program, but I was thrilled for any time I could get out of him.

I couldn't have foreseen the transformation that would take place in my husband! During the course of that workshop he experienced a life-changing epiphany! He finally "got it" that he had a role in the whole fatherhood journey, beyond planting the seed. He became passionate about the father's role in pregnancy and birth and beyond. His entire relationship with the children and I blossomed in ways I cannot even describe. I felt like I had a brand new husband, *masha'Allah*!

When it came time to birth our daughter, he was all for the unassisted homebirth. He not only agreed to it, he looked forward to participating! When her day came, it was my husband who caught her (literally), cleaned up the scene, and took loads of photos. He was so caring and compassionate, *masha'Allah*.

He even wrote a touching memoir of the experience, which is posted on my Saudi Birth Story blog (look up Baby Number Eight). After this experience, I felt so emotionally connected and close to my husband. I really admire how he has grown closer with all of our children as well, *masha'Allah*.

When I began teaching couples, I noticed this same type of transformation taking places in marriages right before my eyes, *masha'Allah*. The Bradley Method® focuses on the husband as coach for his wife and really encourages his full care and support during her pregnancy, labor, and birth.

I truly feel that natural birth and the Bradley Method® are gifts to be given to the expectant parents and their unborn child. However, I soon realized that I can only reach so many women and the American organization just wasn't ready for the explosive global expansion I dream of.

Coming to this reality, I decided to branch out and design my own childbirth preparation materials. I began researching other childbirth methods and quickly found new pieces to the natural childbirth puzzle in Active Birth, by Janet Balakas in the UK. I also saw a great need to bring out the miracles of *Qur'an* and consider culturally sensitive issues to the program.

I cannot express enough my deep gratitude to the American Academy of Husband-Coached Childbirth® and The Bradley Method® for their role in my own births and training as a Childbirth Educator and Doula. They have truly given me the springboard for <u>AMANI Birth</u>. May *Allah* bless this journey and provide many women the best from it and protect them from any harm. *AMEEN*!

WHAT IS AMANI?

AMANI Birth is all about assisting expectant mothers who wish to birth naturally. AMANI Girls is all about advocating programs that motivate preteen and teen girls to live an active lifestyle while focusing on good nutrition with an *Islamic* foundation. In English AMANI Birth and AMANI Girls stands for:

Assisting	**and**	**Advocating**
Mothers for		**Motivation**
Active		**Activity**
Natural		**Nutrition and**
Instinctive		**Islam for**
Birth		**Girls**

The acronyms say it all. In Arabic AMANI means "wishes." When we refer to AMANI in Arabic, we say, "*AMANI lil Welada Tabiaya*," which means, "Wishes for Natural Birth," or "*AMANI lil Banaat*," which means, "Wishes for Girls," which both also say it all. In the context of this text, we will focus on AMANI Birth.

When we speak of "natural" birth, we mean a birth in which the mother is prepared, educated, supported and encouraged to birth without the interference of medicines, medical procedures, or any other unnatural influences. The AMANI concept believes that birthing naturally means more than the reference to how the baby exited the mother's body (birth canal or abdominal surgery). Having said that, <u>AMANI Birth</u> honors the birth experience itself as a natural, sacred act of worship and a display of trust in our Creator, *Allah (SWT)*.

This does not mean she births alone. In fact, we encourage the careful observance of experienced birthing professionals. It simply means that the birthing professionals she chooses are ones who support her all throughout her pregnancy and who trust in the Creator and HIS design of the female body to carry, birth, and feed our babies.

It is our goal to grow the <u>AMANI Birth</u> team to include a huge network of natural birth professionals. These professionals will include <u>AMANI Birth</u> Childbirth Educators, <u>AMANI Birth</u> Certified Doulas, and Certified <u>AMANI Birth</u> Friendly Midwives or Doctors, *in sha' Allah*. <u>AMANI Births</u> can take place in any location. In the future, we hope to evolve the <u>AMANI Birth</u> concept into a certification for <u>AMANI Birth</u> Friendly Hospitals and start a string of free standing <u>AMANI Birth</u> Centers, *insha'Allah*. But even so, an <u>AMANI Birth</u> can take place anywhere from home to hospital or any place in between.

The concept of the <u>AMANI Birth</u> professionals' network is to assist women through awareness, education, preparation and encouragement so that they can prepare themselves to birth the way that women have naturally and instinctively done for thousands of years, *insha'Allah*.

In short, an <u>AMANI Birth</u> is an empowering, natural, non-medicated birth with the woman at the center of the event and the birth attendants supporting and encouraging her all along the way, intervening only if true complications arise.

PART ONE – <u>ASSISTING</u>

In the *Qur'an*, *Allah* clearly tells us to worship only HIM and to seek <u>Assistance</u> from only HIM.

> *"Thee (alone) we worship; Thee alone we ask for help." [Qur'an 1:5]*

HE has perfectly designed and created our bodies to carry, birth, and feed our babies, *subhan'Allah*. But somewhere along the line, women have lost trust in the design of their bodies. Dare I say, that in doing so, we have missed the mark in worshiping *Allah* through trusting and seeking HIM for help in our births? Instead, we are placing our unquestioning trust in the medical industry for "help."

Birth is a beautiful and mysterious journey to be experienced as a worship of trust in *Allah*. Unfortunately, it is often viewed as a traumatic emergency. This is due in part to the sensationalism of modern media. This is further complicated by the over interference of well-intentioned birth attendants, who rush to intervene, in what should most often be a completely natural event.

Additionally, when birthing women moved from their homes and communities into hospitals, *"caring midwives and family birth companions did not go with them,"* (Ina May Gaskin). Tragically, young women lost the opportunity to observe and understand birth. What's more, women in labor lost the caring guidance of their loving and trusted elders to <u>Assist</u>, encourage, and guide them through the emotional and physical challenges of birth.

Birth is a natural and primal event that every woman should be able to conquer. To do so she needs encouragement to tune into her body, trust it and the Creator who designed it, and let instincts take over. However, with our social conditioning to behave "civilized" at all times, coupled with the myriad of distractions and interventions forced in the hospital setting, many women have difficulty letting go of their inhibitions to birth naturally.

Our goal is to return to a culture where women are safe and supported during this most vulnerable, yet empowering time of their lives. To surrender to birth and trust *Allah*, women need emotional support, understanding, and security. This type of <u>*Assistance*</u> is the goal of anyone accompanying an <u>AMANI Birthing</u> Mother.

CHAPTER 1

History of Medical Birth Attendants

Obstetric Care

Obstetrics is the branch of medicine pertaining to pregnancy, labor, and birth. If we look at the word "obstetrics," we find it comes from the Latin word *obstare*, meaning "to stand by." However, in today's birthing culture, obstetric practices have deviated from "standing by" to "dominating women with medical interventions." Many of these interventions are not only unnecessary but are in fact harmful.

The AMANI Birth model encourages obstetric care by qualified midwives or doctors, but discourages obstetric dominance. There was a well-known obstetrician in the United States, Dr. Robert A. Bradley, whose timeless quote in the book Husband-Coached Childbirth, mirrors the AMANI Birth philosophy regarding birth attendants,

"An obstetrician should have a broad rear end and the good sense to sit calmly on it and let nature take its course."

This is not to say that 100% of women can birth completely naturally. We are indeed grateful for obstetric procedures that rescue women and babies when true physical complications arise. However, the vast majority of women can attain an AMANI Birth when they are educated and prepared, insha'Allah. This education and preparation is at the core of every AMANI Birth experience.

The Birth of Obstetrics

The field of obstetric medicine was born, in part, by the work of a French doctor, Dr. François Mauriceau. In 1668 he published *Traité des maladies des femmes grosses, et de celles qui sont accouchées (The Diseases of Women with Child)*. His inspiration to observe women during birth was a result of the tragic loss of his own sister and unborn child during her first birth at the age of twenty.

One of the things he became known for was the introduction of the "French Position" for labor and birth. This bed ridden, reclining position permitted him to more easily observe the patient. Due to the position giving doctors ease in performing medical interventions and procedures, its use quickly spread in Europe and North America.

It was most likely his desire to make good observations of what happens during birth that prompted him to put women on their backs with their legs open. I'm sure it was unbeknownst to him that this is the absolute worst physiological position to birth a baby. Regardless, this simple change affected birthing culture forever, as the role of women in their own births was transformed from instinctual birth-giver, using upright movement for labor and birth, to the passive, back-lying, medical patient that we still see today.

Today's Medicalized Births

As the medical community took over birth, obstetricians became the prevalent birthing attendants. There would be nothing wrong with this model of care if they were trained in birth **normality** first and foremost. But the reality is that obstetricians are skilled surgeons, trained in **abnormality**.

What's worse, many medical birth attendants have never seen a completely active, natural, instinctive birth and some even fear it! Additionally, few have the time to provide the emotional support needed to _Assist_ a woman in natural birth.

Medical school training and hospital protocols and procedures have taught doctors and maternity workers to administer routine interventions to speed and control labor, which can subsequently cause the various complications they are so skilled at managing. What women don't realize is had they foregone the interventions to start with, the skilled lifesaving techniques used to rescue them would likely not have been necessary in the first place!

In Marsden Wagner's Book, _Born in the USA_, he makes a valid point about the troubles of medicalized birth when he quotes a World Health Organization (WHO) statement,

> **"By medicalizing birth, i.e. separating a woman from her own environment and surrounding her with strange people using strange machines to do strange things to her in an effort to _Assist_ her, the woman's state of mind and body is so altered that her way of carrying through this intimate act must also be altered and the state of the baby born must equally be altered. The result is that it is no longer possible to know what births would have been like before these manipulations. Most health care providers no longer know what 'non-medicalized' birth is. The entire modern obstetric and neonatological literature is essentially based on observations of 'medicalized' birth." World Health Organization**

CHAPTER 2

AMANI Birth Attendants

Because the current culture of birth is so medicalized, expectant mothers must be good birth consumers. Sometimes it takes visits to several birth attendants before you're able to find one that you feel confident will support your birthing preferences. Unfortunately, too many times prenatal promises can turn out to be mere lip service with no real intention to fulfill birth requests.

The Vision

This is where we hope the future Certified AMANI Birth Friendly Midwives or Doctors will come in. We plan to have a set criterion for this certification that will give assurance to women that the professionals holding such distinction are aware of the AMANI Birth vision of birth and are dedicated and proven to support women in their AMANI Birth plans, *in sha' Allah*.

The Reality

Until then, women must be prepared to advocate for themselves and their babies to birth with trust in the way *Allah (SWT)* has created us. During the most vulnerable and submissive event of their lives, this is the last thing any woman should have to do! It is mentally and emotionally exhausting to keep your guard while coping with the important and noble work of birthing.

Home Births

For those women who live in regions where home birth is supported, count your blessings! If you are able to stay healthy and low risk, home birth with a qualified birth attendant has been proven to be at least as safe, if not safer than hospital birth and is worth considering.

This writing is not meant to be a home birth versus hospital birth debate. In fact, we maintain that an AMANI Birth should be available to all women, no matter the birthplace.

However, if you would like to explore the research into the safety of home-birth see Outcomes of Planned Home Birth with Registered Midwife Versus Planned Hospital Birth with Midwife or Physician from the *Canadian Medical Association Journal*, which has a commentary and detailed list of resource links at the end of the article.

For an excellent read about the safety of planned home birth with a wealth of resources, I recommend the article Fish Can't See Water: The Need To Humanize Birth by Marsden Wagner, MD, MSPH, published in the *International Journal of Gynecology & Obstetrics*. Dr. Wagner retired as head of Maternal and Child Health for the European Office of the World Health Organization (WHO) and continues to serve as a consultant for WHO. He is well known amongst natural birth advocates for his public support of midwifery, midwives, and homebirth.

Unfortunately, many of the families reading this book won't have such accessible options in their local communities. For them, it is especially important that they take the time to get educated about their options and exercise conviction and determination to strive for the best birth experience for mother and baby, whether they choose to navigate the hospital birthing system or birth unassisted at home.

The Hope

However, I am pleased to say that there are physicians out there, like gems amongst the rocks, supporting and trusting women's desires and abilities to birth naturally. I have the pleasure to know two such doctors personally. Both have become childbirth educators in addition to attending births as they have seen the need to educate women. They both understand the value of the husband's role in supporting his wife emotionally during pregnancy and labor and encourage fathers to participate in the births of their children.

One is Dr. Fernando Molina, MD of Venezuela. Dr. Fernando has been serving as a childbirth educator and is certified in water births. He has been attending homebirths, with his wife serving as doula, since 1998. His passion for and understanding of the needs of women during labor and birth are inspiring.

The second is Dr. Hanna Abo Kassem, OB of Egypt. Dr. Hanna became acquainted with natural birth and began to tear down the walls of fear and medical dominance in birth in her private practice in 2010. Her recent transformation from "recommending elective Cesarean" to "teaching natural birth" took place before my eyes and gives me hope for other medical birth attendants who are oppressed by their medical training which mostly focuses on protocols and abnormality, despite birth being completely normal in the majority of cases.

Sadly, as Dr. Hanna confided in me, medical training rarely, if ever, covers birth as a natural physiological event in a woman's life. In fact, she had never even seen a completely natural birth when I met her, despite being a practicing obstetrician for over fifteen years! Coincidentally, as I'm writing this, Dr. Hanna has attended her very first homebirth, *masha'Allah*!

This news gives me a glimmer of hope in our aim to reach other medical professionals with the training and information needed to change the culture of birth from medical dominance to maternal choice and respect. I really don't fault medical professionals. They are simply following their instincts; which are programmed from early on in their careers to look for problems and constantly introduce medical interventions. After all, they are trained to "do something," "anything," not just sit and observe. It really takes patience, confidence, and emotional stamina to serve the role of lifeguard while encouraging the woman through, what may be the most emotionally physically and challenging, yet rewarding event of her life.

AMANI Birth Attendants

Our vision of AMANI Birth Attendants are those who:

- Willingly support mothers in natural birth

- Display inner confidence and trust in *Allah's* wisdom and design of the mother's body to birth naturally

- Apply patient observation, rather than rushed intervention

- Strive to provide the privacy and respect needed to achieve the primal state of birth

- Never put their own schedule ahead of *Allah's* decree

- Set aside their own comforts for the comfort and ease of the birth

- Let go of their position at "center stage" and hand the honors to mother and baby

- Listen to mothers and *Assist* them to achieve the experiences they desire

- Treat mothers as individuals, foregoing the assembly line approach of routine protocols and procedures

- Keep an open mind to birth, which is outside the textbook model approach

- Surrender to the reality that they are not in control of birth, only careful observers and patient lifeguards, only getting wet when someone is truly drowning

There is a saying, *"Where there is a will, there is a way."* AMANI Birth Attendants respect the time, effort, and preparations taken by AMANI Birth parents. They look for ways to implement and support their birth plans to ensure safe and satisfying birth experiences for mothers, babies, and families. They recognize the birth of a child as the birth of a family. Perhaps most importantly, they honor the birth experience, and precious moments that follow. They recognize that these precious moments will forever affect the character and personality of the baby and serve as the foundation that families are built on.

Calling All Birth Attendants

For those medical professionals who stand for women's rights to birth naturally and trust *Allah's* design for that purpose, we applaud you. In fact, we'd like to meet you and discover your journey to "the other side." We would like to work with you to help us build the AMANI Birth Certification and be among the first to hold this designation.

If you are a medical student, midwife, or experienced doctor who would like to explore more, we invite you to sift through the pages of this book with an open mind and an open heart towards truly *Assisting* women and children in birth, rather than taking over for them.

CHAPTER 3

Childbirth Education

At the core of AMANI Birth is education. In fact, in this section, *Assisting*, it may well be the most important piece of the proverbial jigsaw puzzle of natural birth. We truly feel that by seeking education about the journey through pregnancy, labor and birth, women are *Assisting* themselves to understand the process and the choices they are obliged to make. It's also important to realize that by not making any decisions, women make the boldest and possibly worst decision of all: that is the decision to turn their body over to the doctor like a car to a mechanic.

History of Childbirth Education

In the past, childbirth was a community event. Neighboring women and extended family, both up and down the generational ladder, typically came together to *Assist* laboring mothers. Young girls witnessed birth and had knowledge of the process long before it was their turn to deliver. Birth was considered a natural event and childbirth education was an informal passing of knowledge from one generation to the next.

Unfortunately, when childbirth moved into the hospitals, the chain of knowledge was lost. Often times an expectant mother's first view of birth was her own. Women returned from hospital delivery rooms telling the horrors and pains they endured. Birth became an extremely medicalized event filled with terrifying mystery, fear, and anxiety.

British Obstetrician, Dr. Grantly Dick-Read, began to speak out against medical interventions in childbirth in the 1930s. His philosophy was based on the belief that childbirth is a natural event and that much of the pain experienced came from doctor interference, coupled with the fears and ensuing tensions surrounding birth. He authored the well-known book *Childbirth Without Fear*, which became an international best seller in the 1940s. His work sparked public interest in "*natural birth*," a term he coined to describe birthing with as little intervention from obstetricians as possible.

French Obstetrician, Dr. Fernand Lamaze, promoted a hypnotic approach to birth based indirectly on the work of Russian Physiologist, Ivan Pavlov. He authored *Painless Childbirth: The Lamaze Method* in 1956. From this work, childbirth education was born. Subsequently, attending childbirth classes became popular and widespread amongst women in the West. However, The Lamaze Method has branched off in many directions over the years. Often times it is taught in hospitals and is diluted by focus on protocols and procedure, thus preparing women for what to expect and encouraging them to be "good patients," rather than understanding the normal process of unhindered labor and birth. At its core, the Lamaze Method is a fabulous source of childbirth education and support.

American Obstetrician, Dr. Robert A. Bradley, was inspired by the work of both predecessors. Having grown up on a farm, he had witnessed many animals laboring calmly and naturally. During his study of obstetrics, he was astounded to see women in the hospital setting being "delivered" by a series of medical interventions in an out-of-control-drugged state. He challenged the medical model of labor and piloted childbirth classes designed to teach women to imitate the natural deliveries he had seen by animals. He was the first to introduce husbands *Assisting* their wives in the delivery room, which gained widespread popularity in the West and forever changed the birthing culture. In 1965, he authored *Husband-Coached Childbirth*. From this came the formation of the American Academy of Husband-Coached Childbirth®, which he founded with his patient, Marjie Hathaway and her husband Jay. Together they developed a twelve-week series of formal classes teaching couples about the process of pregnancy, labor, and birth in order to know what to expect and to prepare for it. The Bradley Method® also encourages good nutrition and exercise to remain healthy and low-risk during pregnancy. Dr. Bradley wrote that birth was an athletic event that required physical, mental, and emotional preparation on the part of a woman, coached by her husband. In the Bradley Method®, total relaxation is the key to hard labor and expectant parents are taught the importance of avoiding drugs at any time during pregnancy, labor, and birth unless there are serious complications where their benefits outweigh the risks. Parents who take Bradley® classes prepare birth plans and take responsibility for the decisions made during their births. They typically shop around for a birth attendant and birthplace that they feel will support their birth plan and thus become "good birth consumers."

South African Childbirth Educator, Janet Balaskas, entered the birth scene in the 1970s and made history in the 1980s in the United Kingdom with the introduction of "Active Birth," a term she coined to describe freedom of movement and upright positions during labor and birth. She has written many books including *Active Birth* in 1983. She challenged the obstetric model of maternity care and advocates for women to get off their back as "passive patients" and to be "upright givers of birth" instead. Her public organization of women in favor of her philosophy literally changed birthing culture in the UK and places women at the center of their pregnancy, labor, and birth.

AMANI Birth, although written by an American, originates in Saudi Arabia, the birthplace of *Islam*. AMANI Birth, the book, childbirth education program, doula training, and vision for birth centers, has been inspired by all of the preceding childbirth education pioneers. However, trust in *Allah* as our Creator and perfect Designer of birth as a form of *Islamic* worship is missing in all of the aforementioned childbirth education methods.

I am far from an *Islamic* scholar, however, I find that in researching *Qur'an*, *Hadeeth*, and *Sunnah*, there are only a few specific references to birth with regards to Maryam's/Mary's (*Alayhas-Salam*) delivery of Isa/Jesus (*Alayhis-Salām*) and a few general acknowledgment of the pains and burdens of birth and breastfeeding. There are, however, references to hardships and illnesses that can be applied to birth as well. Using common sense it's easy to infer that natural birth, that is birth without medicinal pain relief, must be *Sunnah*, given that such interference didn't exist at the time of the

Prophet Muhammad (*Sallallaahu 'alayhi wa sallam*) over fourteen hundred years ago.

As a former Certified Bradley® Childbirth Educator and Lecturer, I am particularly endeared to the Bradley Method®. Although I am a strong believer in Dr. Bradley's philosophies and husbands as labor coaches, I find there to be some conflict within Arab society to the participation of fathers at birth, although this is slowly changing, *alhamdulillah*. Additionally, the hospital-birthing climate in Egypt, UAE, Kuwait, and Saudi Arabia mirrors the medical model of the Untied States with an added dominance that can overpower even the most prepared natural birthing mother.

I first considered introducing the Bradley Method® to the Middle East on a grand scale. However, as I have come to know more about the Arab culture and extremely difficult hospital birthing climate that mothers often face here, I realized there needs to be a more dynamic and culturally sensitive approach to childbirth education in this region than is currently offered in Husband-Coached Childbirth®. Of course, I can't help but incorporate many of the valuable principles I learned from my training in the Bradley Method® into <u>AMANI Birth</u>.

<u>AMANI Birth</u> has evolved from the inspiration of the many pioneers before it and is propelled by the unique needs of our *Muslim* sisters in the Middle East and beyond. It's time for an *Islamic* chapter of childbirth education to be written, one that honors our Creator through trust in birth and that welcomes fathers, yet empowers women. <u>AMANI Birth</u> is <u>*Assisting* Mothers for Active, Natural, Instinctive Birth</u>.

Only YOU Can Birth YOUR Baby

If there was one thing I wish women could understand, it's the fact that no one can breathe for you, live for you, die for you, or birth for you. You are on your own. In fact, birthing completely alone might seem scary, but honestly, if you tune into your body, you have all the skill and know-how you need to birth your baby.

That may sound extreme. Please do not mistake the message. I'm not saying you must or should birth alone. But I am saying that you have the control, power, and intuition to birth. I am simply opening up the dialogue of empowerment and capability that *Allah (SWT)* has given to every woman.

Current Birthing Culture

The current culture of birth is fear based. Sadly, our medical communities, our media, and even our own mothers often instill that birth is an impending emergency looming in the future. We convey the message that birth must somehow be "managed" by a professional and that all mothers and babies need to be "rescued."

Generations of Births

I must speak out to challenge this paradigm. For those who take time to ponder, you can't overlook the fact that the majority of women can birth, just as Maryam/Mary (*Alayhas-Salam*) mother of Isa/Jesus (*Alayhis-Salām*) and the generations of women since Hawwa/Eve (*Alayhas-Salam*) have done. That is completely instinctually, without medications, or medical interference.

Importance of Education

On my Saudi Birth Story blog, I wrote an article, "Who's to Blame?". In this article I discuss the woman's responsibility to get educated and take control of her birth:

Who's to Blame?

I WRITE a lot about the benefits of having a natural, non-medicated birth. I tell you that I respect doctors while also seeming to "*blame*" them for the many "unnecessary" medical interventions that often take over the birth process. Well it's time to put things into perspective and look at the bigger picture.

Please note that this article is totally based on my opinion, which no doubt weighs heavy on the side of natural birth.

First, I want to acknowledge that there is a word in the English language to describe an illness or adverse condition in a patient that is **caused** by the medical treatment they receive. The fact that we even have such a word saddens me. _Iatrogenic_ is this word that describes adverse conditions brought at the hands of the doctor, the one we rely on for our care, our health, and our bodies - usually with complete trust and without much question.

Although I contend that there are many problems that occur during labor and birth that are _iatrogenic_, I do not believe that our trusted doctors intentionally harm us. In fact, in most instances, I'd venture to say that they truly believe that what they are doing is in our best interest.

One simple, seemingly harmless example is the routine use of glucose IV. It is often used to prevent dehydration and gives doctors _"peace of mind"_ that a line is running to the vein, "just in case a need arises for a higher medicinal administration."

I agree that it is imperative to prevent dehydration during labor and birth. Dehydration can cause very serious complications and it is reasonable for the doctor to want to safeguard his patient from these complications. However, we must consider that the unnecessary _"routine"_ of administering glucose intravenously alters the blood sugar levels of mother and baby. The IV line itself also limits the mother's mobility during labor and birth (a time when movement is paramount).

To top it off, it was also noted in the July, 1984 edition of _The American Journal of Medicine_ (Volume 77), **_"...rapid increases in circulating glucose levels produce a decrease in the ability of normal persons to tolerate pain."_** Regardless of the other issues involved with unnecessary IVs, the simple possibility that it could reduce my ability to tolerate pain is reason enough for me to refuse it. Personally, I think childbirth is painful enough!

So what's wrong with drinking water? This is the natural way to stay hydrated. Even in the English translation of the _Qur'an_ (Y. Ali 19:26) it says, **_"So eat and drink and cool (thine) eye,"_** referring to providing relief to Mary whilst in labor with Jesus (_Alayhis-Salām_). Clearly, _Allah_ was offering water to drink, not a glucose IV to Mary during her labor. If it were good enough for Mary, I'd say it's good enough for me!

As for the *"open line to the vein, just in case,"* a capped off IV catheter can be inserted and accessed quickly enough in the event of an emergency. But frankly, I'd prefer there not be an *"open line"* that gives such ready access to drugs entering my veins while I'm not looking or have not been properly informed of what's being given and why.

I could ramble on and on about unnecessary medical protocols and elective medications. I could site several examples about medical procedures interfering with the natural process of birth. I could explain how interfering with one medical intervention increases the likelihood for the next higher intervention until finally you're having an "emergency" cesarean. Instead, I want to discuss the reasons why I believe our trusted doctors introduce these things to us in the first place.

- It is what they have been trained to do. No, not to harm us or to cause us iatrogenic injury, but to medically manage our labors, rather than patiently watching them happen. Let's face it, they paid a lot of money and put a lot of time into their medical education. That education has taught them how to manage abnormality, although the vast majority of women would experience complete normality in their labor and birth, if we just left them alone and let nature take its course.

- Sadly, most women are not trained or prepared to handle natural childbirth. Women often come in requesting that first intervention (pain medication) which sets off an entire chain of events that, simply put, is not natural and raises risks for both her and the baby.

- Along the same lines, women do not take the time to educate themselves about the physiology of pregnancy, labor, and birth. Therefore they do not know the intrinsic behaviors needed to work with their bodies at this important time. <u>Honestly, a woman uneducated in the way her body works during labor and birth is her own worst enemy.</u>

- Because the majority of women are not prepared, doctors seldom see a calm, confident woman who knows how to cope with her labor and birth without the aid of drugs or other medical interventions.

21

Most doctors and other obstetric professionals have rarely, if ever, witnessed a completely natural, non-medicated birth. From their perspective, normality is actually the abnormality and abnormality is the "*norm.*"

- Lastly, doctors have a job to do. That job requires them to come to work at all hours of the day and night. It is much more convenient for the doctor to take over the birth process, even to the point of performing elective cesarean surgeries to make it all fit their own personal schedules. So what's wrong with this if it's what the mother wants? Ahh, the answers to that one, I'll save for another post.

From my perspective, it's the mother who's to blame for the *iatrogenic* problems in childbirth. That's right, I said it, "**The mother herself is to blame for adverse conditions brought on at the hands of her trusted doctor.**" It all boils down to her lack of education and preparation for her own birth.

Every woman has nine months warning that she will be laboring and birthing at some estimated future date. I find it completely irresponsible of her to just hand her body over to her obstetrician like a car to the mechanic. After all, this is her body we're talking about, not to mention her baby!

Bottom line: if you're pregnant, or ever plan to be, get educated, get prepared, and become a responsible birth consumer. Don't just be complacent to the protocols that are designed to manage abnormality. Assume normality until there's some reason not to. Explore your options and make informed decisions about what you want for your labor and birth. Stay flexible and know that things may not go as planned, but I'm here to tell you, nothing goes as planned when there is no plan!

The AMANI Birth Goal

AMANI Birth's goal is to train, certify, and mentor passionate and dedicated Childbirth Educators; who in turn, penetrate local communities to educate, prepare, and *Assist* expectant mothers and anyone they have chosen to accompany them during their labor and birth. Although AMANI Birth is founded for the sake of *Allah* and with *Islamic* trust and worship in mind, it is of benefit to women of any faith who wish to understand how to prepare for natural birth.

Become an AMANI Birth Mother and/or Educator/Doula

To become an AMANI Birth Childbirth Educator/Doula or to locate an Educator/Doula in your area, visit www.amanibirth.com. With *Allah's* will, our educators will *Assist* women across the globe with love for the sake of *Allah* and encouragement to trust *Allah* and HIS perfect design of their bodies during the most vulnerable, yet empowering time in their lives.

CHAPTER 4

Family and Friends as Labor Companions

Birth is more than challenging, hard work; it's the celebration of a new life, a new member of the family and community. It's natural to desire loving support during this trying time, as well as wanting to share the once-in-a-lifetime event with those you love.

I would caution, however, to choose wisely. The people in your labor and birth environment will have an effect on the intensity and ease (or difficulty) of the labor and birth itself. Be sure that your labor companions are prepared for the emotional roller coaster and graphic visuals of labor and birth.

Create the Birth Team

Every witness to the birth should be considered part of the birth team and should understand the process of birth. Everyone in the room should be aware of the mother's birth vision and be committed to supporting and encouraging her through the process, *in sha' Allah*.

The AMANI Birth program has modules specifically designed for labor companions. These modules should be completed by all prospective birth partners, alongside the expectant mother. They will help everyone to understand, not only the process of birth, but also their role in the birth. During classes, participants will discover what the mother visualizes for her birth and what help she needs.

Mother's Choice of Companion(s)

Each woman has a different sense of who they do (or do not) want at their birth. This can be deep rooted by culture, religion, and personal experience. Personally, I feel that the husband makes a great labor companion. After all, birth is a very intimate and vulnerable time and there is no one I need, love, or trust more than my husband. Admittedly, I recognize that this also stems from the influences of American culture; where men are *expected* to be at the birth and are even shunned if they're not.

On the other hand, some women couldn't bear to have their husband's see them in such a vulnerable state. They don't feel they could relax and surrender to the birth if he's watching. Similarly, just as I could not fathom having my mother or sister present (no offense to either of them), some women long for the loving support and comfort that they feel from them.

The point is, think carefully and do not feel obliged to include anyone on the basis of his or her desire to be there or of not wanting to hurt their feelings. At the same time, it is probably not beneficial to force someone to be there who is uncomfortable or resistant to do so (such as a husband).

Family Politics of Birth

It can be very difficult for women who find themselves in a dilemma of having unwelcome persons inviting themselves to the birth. If you are that person, it's important to remember that this is HER birth. Expectant mothers have a lot to deal with in labor and birth and no one should force themselves on her or take offense if she doesn't feel comfortable sharing such an intense and intimate time with them, no matter who they are!

Unfortunately, this can become a matter of family politics and can plant the seeds for discord and hard feelings. Feel free to share this book and point out this section if you feel your family falling prey to hard feelings in this regard.

If you would like to attend someone else's birth, I suggest you offer to be there but end your offer with a statement of understanding in case she may not want you there: **"I'd really love to be with you for your birth. But please don't feel obligated. If you'd like me there, I'll be thrilled; but no offense if not."**

If you are the expectant mother in this situation, do your best to be diplomatic, but follow your instincts. If it doesn't seem right to you to have someone there, tell him or her right away. Don't let it fester and be a source of stress to you. You could say something like, **"Aww, that's so sweet of you. I love your support and care! But to be honest, I'm a little shy and nervous about being watched during birth and would prefer you not be there. I'm sure you understand."** In sha' Allah, the other person will be mature enough not to take offense.

Many Men Resist Birth

Conversely, an expectant mother may feel devastated or let down if the person she really needs or wants is resistant or refuses to be there. This can leave huge emotional scars for the mother and in the relationship. Obviously, this is especially detrimental if that person is her husband.

In fact, my own marriage suffered due to my husband's resistance to attend our first two births together. However, understanding the underlying causes of his reluctance (lack of knowledge and education) helped me through my emotional struggle.

But more importantly, during the pregnancy of our third child he welcomed education about the pregnancy, labor, and birth process, alhamdu-lillah. Through this education he reached an epiphany about his important role during birth. Because of this, he transformed into the loving, caring, birth companion that I needed during the birth of our third child. We experienced a growth and bonding in our marriage and our family due to his transformation that is difficult to describe in words.

On my Saudi Life Motherhood column, I wrote an article, "Husbands at Birth in Saudi." In this article, I discuss the increasing pressure on men to attend births as well as their important role as protector of women. I also address the typical reasons men are reluctant to attend births and acknowledge that some men really shouldn't be there at all. I conclude with the way in which marriages grow stronger when he makes the effort to learn more.

Husbands at Birth in Saudi

IT wasn't until our third birth together that my husband finally "got" his role as labor coach, advocate, and protector over me and our unborn baby. Even so, the first obstetrician we visited in Saudi reacted as if we were from Mars when we asked about his presence in the labor and delivery room. She went so far as to tell us, ***"Birth is no place for husbands! No hospital will ever allow that!"*** She even insinuated that this is the case worldwide!

Obviously, she was not only misinformed (or lying, *astaghfirullah*) about men in hospital delivery rooms, but she didn't realize just whom she was talking to! I quickly shot back, ***"Well you won't be <u>my</u> doctor for delivery, that's for sure!"*** The look of shock on her face was priceless. It was as if, in her mind, I had no other choice, after all I was sitting in **<u>her</u>** clinic for the consult.

Even though I had no intention of birthing with her, I could feel my blood pressure rising during the exchange. The mere thought of this doctor's condescending and dominant manner advising less knowledgeable couples during their pregnancies made my blood boil!

As for my husband, we had reached a plateau with regards to his commitment to supporting me during birth, *alhamdulillah*; but it wasn't his initial or immediate response to the idea. In fact, he wasn't present with me for our first two births.

Like many men all over the world he simply felt clueless and out of place around the idea of birth. He had no idea as to what role he could play or what he could actually **<u>do</u>** to help me during labor and birth. Due to the obscurity of their roles, men are often reluctant to attend. To top that off, men are problem solvers by nature; however, birth is not a problem to be solved; rather, it's an experience to be shared.

Increasing Social Pressure on Men

Like it or not, men are facing more and more pressure to be there for their wives at this important time. There is often hesitance even in Western men, where it is not only customary but also **expected** for husbands to attend birth. Due to the increased influences of Western values in Saudi Arabia, young Saudis are starting to find themselves facing this pressure as well.

It can be particularly disappointing and stressful for Western women married to Saudis (or other non-Westerners) to realize that their husbands may flat out refuse to attend. This can cause marital discord and stress. This is complicated by her status as an expatriate, since she typically does not have her female family members available to her in Saudi for emotional support and accompaniment. As a result, she turns even more desperately to her husband to fulfill that role.

But it's important to note that in addition to the Western influence on Saudi culture, modernization has also deteriorated the traditional extended family bonds and support here as well. Because of this, young Saudi women may not have the female support system of the past generations. It's only natural that she also turns to her husband to fulfill this role, regardless of her traditional culture.

Saudi's Evolving Birth Culture

Irrespective of changing needs and family dynamics, Saudi culture still seems to favor birth as mostly off-limits to husbands. As I noted in State of Birth in Saudi Arabia, my own husband told me during our first pregnancy together, "*In my culture, birth is a woman's thing, you know. Men don't participate like they do in your country.*"

However, the fact that there are a growing number of hospitals in Saudi that do allow the husband into the labor and delivery rooms is a sign of change. Although this is evidence of birthing culture evolution here, Saudi is still behind other nations in fully accepting, or expecting, men to attend the birth of their babies.

To be fair, it's not just Saudi men or Saudi culture that feels this nervous uneasiness around a man's role (or not) in birth. In fact, I'd venture to guess it's quite similar in most Arab cultures, as well as Pakistan, and India, to name just a few. Similarly, just because it has become part of the birthing culture in the West, doesn't mean all Western men are keen to the idea, although the social and cultural pressures on them to participate are great.

Frankly speaking, lack of compassion on the part of some men as well as some extreme phobias around bodily functions/fluids and the like, really do preclude the presence of a few. It truly is not in anyone's best interest to try to force those who are adamantly against it.

But all culture and individual preferences or issues aside, I can tell you that I've witnessed and experienced the benefits of the presence and support of a loving husband at birth. The husband simply being there during her most vulnerable and intense moments provides immeasurable comfort and calm to the laboring woman. Often, as a result, her admiration of him is heightened; as is his loving respect and protective nature for her.

What About Her Mother?

But even for the woman whose husband cannot (or will not) accompany her, she really does need someone (other than the medical staff) to be with her. Then the question arises, "If not him, then who?"

Often times the answer is her mother or her mother-in-law. But many women find this uncomfortable due to the hierarchy of behavior expected when an "elder" is present as well as possible conflicts between the way the older woman birthed and the birth preferences of the younger (especially if the older woman's births were medically dominated and the younger is committed to natural birth...or vice versa). Another option is to hire a doula (see What is a Doula?). This is often a much better choice than her own mother or mother-in-law.

Birth is a very intimate event. Personally speaking, there simply is no one I trust more to share such a vulnerable and private time, than the father. No offense to my mother, who I love dearly, but I would not feel comfortable with her in attendance at my birth. But that's just ME.

Men are Protectors of Women

Women really do need to be protected during birth, especially in a hospital setting. This has nothing to do with hospitals in Saudi. I'm speaking regardless of the country. It has more to do with her level of vulnerability during labor and birth.

I do recognize that birth can be terrifying to men. But stop and think about this, if it's frightening to HIM, how much more so is it to the woman? Shouldn't he, as her protector, be brave enough to at least be there with her as she goes through it?

Protecting women is what men really do well, *masha'Allah*. For men are truly protectors of women. Once a husband realizes that his wife is going to need him during this very vulnerable time, he "gets it" that this is **HIS** role and no one else's!

"Men are the protectors...of women..." [Qur'an 4:34]

Men's Discomfort Around Birth

I can also understand, however, that men don't want to see the one they love in pain, especially without the ability to FIX it. This is compounded by the knowledge that he was part of the cause! Additionally, most men can't stand being useless or feeling clueless about what's going on. With birth as an unknown *"woman thing,"* they just lack the confidence and knowledge to *Assist*.

The best response to this is for couples to make joint efforts to get educated and prepare for the birth (physically, emotionally, and mentally). Childbirth education is the ideal setting, but it can also be through reading and research. Such active preparation eases fears, gives both parties confidence, and teaches each what to do and when.

Stronger Marriages

I have had the pleasure and honor to witness husbands discovering their roles, including practical things they can do to actually help their laboring wife. With this discovery, most men transition into enthused labor coaches and advocates for their wives and babies. Even for the husband who only commits to spending her early labor with her, then plans to see her to the door for the birth, there is a significant amount of time that he will want to know how he can help her. Not to mention, if there are complications, he is the one that will be looked to for making medical decisions. Having some knowledge of the birth process will give him greater confidence to fulfill this role on behalf of his wife and baby as well, *in sha' Allah*.

For men who may be "on the fence" about whether or not to step up to the plate as labor coach, just consider how much it means to your wife. For her, taking classes (or researching together) confirms her husband's commitment to her and really proves that he cares for her and loves her. I can attest to the ten-fold strengthening of marriages that inevitably results, *masha'Allah*.

It honestly is heartwarming to watch, as couples grow closer together through the course of childbirth classes. What's even more beautiful is realizing that as they become confident in their abilities, it applies not only to birthing together, but to raising their new family together as well, *masha'Allah*.

She Needs You There

If you are that person who is needed and wanted by the expectant mother, but feel resistant to be there, I'd suggest you explore your feelings and discuss it openly with the mother. It's important to realize that she will likely feel rejected and uncared for and this has the potential to cause problems between you that go far beyond the birth. She needs to know that you really care for her, despite your lack of enthusiasm for attending the birth.

Usually this applies to husbands. I find that most men, across the board (regardless of race, culture, or religion), are not as keen to playing the role of birth partner as his wife would like. In fact, while teaching childbirth classes I found that the husbands usually attended the first class after the incessant pleadings of their wives. Most often their first question to me was, **"Do I have to attend ALL the classes?"**

Husbands Need Educational Support

As addressed in the article above, it usually boils down to the male nature. Men simply don't like to feel ignorant about things and they also don't like not knowing what to do. Once they attend classes they are usually eager to attend the birth and feel a sense of obligation to protect their wife and baby. Husbands truly make the best advocates for their laboring wives.

In fact, I believe that providing the father with this education is as important as the expectant mother herself. Even if he has no intention of witnessing the birth, it is he who will be turned to for making important medical decisions, especially in the unlikely event of an emergency. Understanding the process and terminology of birth is imperative for him to competently handle that role.

He should also know what his wife will go through in order to better understand his role in supporting her in preparing for birth during the pregnancy period. After all, no one has greater interest in the health and welfare and outcome of the birth than the mother, baby, and father. Similarly, no one loves the mother and baby like the father. He too will live with the lifelong consequences of the mother's preparation (or lack thereof) and her decisions (or lack of them) for her labor and birth.

Mother's Pain Becomes Loved One's Discomfort

One other consideration about family and friends as labor companions is the emotional toil that birth takes on all people involved. It is often harder on the mother's loved ones to see her in pain than the pain itself is on her. This point was nicely demonstrated in Sarah Buckley's book, _Gentle Birth, Gentle Mothering_, where she wrote about the photos taken immediately after her birth:

"My face in those early photos has no lingering hint of pain, but Nicholas looks drawn and exhausted, reminding me that the role of birth supporter is also enormous, but without the ability to release the energy and fear through noise and movement."

One of the AMANI Birth goals during the *Assisting* modules is to prepare the birth companions to cope with their own feelings of fear and emotional discomfort that come from seeing the mother experience the pains of labor and birth. Once they realize the necessity of the pain to the experience, and understand the movements and noises associated with it, they recognize that what they are witnessing are actually coping mechanisms for mother. This makes them better equipped to encourage her to let go of her inhibitions and surrender to her instinctual needs to make the primal expressions and sounds that help her through.

Men's Growth

I'd like to follow-up my lament about my Saudi husband's lack of support with the heartwarming and amazing change in his stance by our third birth. He has learned more about pregnancy, labor, and birth than most pregnant women, *masha'Allah*.

With that knowledge came the understanding of what women are up against in the medical model of birth. He used to believe it was okay to just send her behind the double doors and the doctors would take care of everything. He never knew that there were a myriad of decisions to be made, each creating a twist and turn towards the final outcome. Even more, he didn't realize that in the absence of support, his wife would become vulnerable to many unnecessary interventions, which often result in iatrogenic (doctor caused) complications that increase the risks of birth as well as cause emotional and physical birth trauma and injury to both mother and child.

Once he became aware of the realities, he experienced an epiphany that transformed him from "indifferent and distant from the birthing process" to "protective, caring, supportive, and involved guardian." He rushed to the duty of protecting me during our third birth and even went so far as to support my decision to birth at home, without any medical _Assistance_.

I cannot begin to tell you how bonded he is to Amani, the daughter he literally "caught." Even so, AMANI Birth does not advocate nor teach unassisted birthing. It was our personal choice and we were comfortable with the perceived risks. We felt confident in our decision to do birth alone and can identify with others who come to the same decision. But please understand that this was not something we decided lightly and it was after my becoming exasperated with the emotional and mental turmoil of repeated hospital births.

Men Protect Their Families

His transformation did not happen overnight; however, it is so profound that I am happy to tell you that he became a better, more caring and involved husband and father to all our children, _alhamdulillah_. Our marriage became closer and stronger when this stubborn, Arab man realized his duty to protect and support us on a level he had never realized before.

> _"Men are the protectors and maintainers of women, because Allah has given the one more (strength) than the other..."_ [Qur'an 4:34]

Alhamdulillah, this strength comes shining through at birth, when a woman is in her weakest state and most vulnerable to outside influences and interventions. The husband truly does make the best protector and guardian, in my opinion, but more important than my opinion is what will work for each individual couple.

Just be sure that every person in the labor and delivery room is ready to encourage and has unwavering faith in the mother in labor. Love, safety, and encouragement are what she really needs, regardless who it comes from.

CHAPTER 5

Professional Labor Companions

More and more parents are turning to the help and support of professional labor companions. These caring women are usually not medically trained, although they are trained in birth and have a vast range of experience. Most AMANI Birth Educators are also certified as AMANI Birth Doulas. So what exactly is a "*Doula*" and what do they do?

Description of Doulas

On my Saudi Life Motherhood column, I wrote an article, "What is a Doula?" At the time the article was written, AMANI Birth had not begun training doulas yet. Fortunately, by the time you read this there should be AMANI Birth doulas around the world to choose from, *in sha' Allah*. In this article, I describe the role and duties of a professional labor companion:

What is a Doula?

DOULA services for labor/birth and the postpartum period are becoming more and more popular and well known worldwide. In fact, they are becoming commonplace in many developed nations such as the UK, USA, Switzerland, and Australia. Even in the UAE there are growing numbers of doulas available, *masha'Allah*. I'm also aware of doulas in Qatar, Oman, Bahrain, and Egypt, although the numbers are far less.

However, the concept seems to be fairly new here in Saudi. Many of my regular readers are aware that I am a doula, but I've only met two other doulas in Riyadh. Of course there may be others out there that I just haven't had the pleasure to meet. (I'd love to hear from any and invite their communication.)

So what is a doula and who needs one?

A doula is a woman who provides non-medical support during pregnancy, labor, birth, and the postpartum period (recovery time after birth). They usually have training and experience in childbirth, although they are not medically trained. Typically they will meet with the pregnant woman several times to help inform her of her choices and what to expect in birth. The doula will take the time to know her client's desires for her birth and will encourage her to write a birth plan and provide tips for effectively communicating her wishes to her medical birth team.

Some doulas also offer some form of formal or informal childbirth preparation training as well. It is also common for the doula to stay with the mother for a short time after delivery to ensure a good start with feeding and caring for her new baby, as well as provide _Assistance_ in the mother's care. Many doulas will make house visits during the postpartum period or may even provide comprehensive postpartum services which would include staying at the woman's residence to help to care for the newborn, new mother, and pick up the slack in the household chores (cooking, cleaning, laundry, caring for elder children, etc.).

The duties and roles of the doula vary from case to case. What is wanted and needed by the woman and how the doula can fill these needs, is one of the many things they will decide upon during the pregnancy visits. This individualized attention and care can rarely be offered by any other child-birth professional.

In the hospital setting, the nurses, midwives, and doctors are busy attending to many patients and other duties. The doctor may not even be the same doctor she has had visits with during her pregnancy. Regardless, he or she often times does not come until it is time for the actual delivery of the baby. By this time the woman has usually spent a significant amount of time at the hospital in labor. The laboring woman can expect occasional checks during her labor, but most likely will not have someone from the hospital staff at her side the whole time (unless there are serious complications and she is being closely monitored). One major benefit of having a doula is that the laboring woman (and her family) can be assured they will not be left to labor alone. This is also a benefit to the medical staff as the patient and family are usually less needy or dependent on them for every small detail of the labor.

Having a doula can also provide a great relief of stress. This is especially true for the father, who may be the only other support person to attend the labor. In many cases the father (and mother for that matter) is unfamiliar with the birth process, medical protocols, and is simply at a loss as to what he can do to help. (Of course I recommend all parents take childbirth preparation classes, which help to alleviate this situation.)

Additionally, since the doula is not usually an employee of the hospital, parents often trust the doula to provide unbiased information. Parents should be informed, however, that although the doula may be able to explain complicated medical terminology, she should not make decisions nor give specific advice about medical matters. She is a good source of information based on her experience, but she remains neutral in her involvement of medical matters and reminds the mother that it is her responsibility to make all decisions and to work with the medical team in doing so.

It is the doula's role to support the woman as well as other family members who may be participating in the birth. It is her goal to help the woman have a safe and satisfying birth experience based on what each individual woman desires. This can be especially important to women who are residing away from extended family or who are foreigners in the country of the birth. These women typically will not have the traditional support of other, experienced mothers from their own family (mother, sister, aunt, etc.) to guide them through. The doula fills this gap by providing an important support throughout the pregnancy, birth, and postpartum time.

Even if the husband (or other relative) will attend the birth, a doula can provide support to the entire family. She encourages the husband and suggests things that he can do to help his laboring wife. She supports his role and does not replace his participation at the birth. Her ultimate goal is a good birth experience and positive family bonding of all members of the family through the miraculous experience of birth.

In an era where birth has become a process of medical management, a doula can _Assist_ the family in understanding the natural process and help them to have confidence in it.

Although the doula supports the woman's choices regarding the use (or not) of medical interventions (pain relief, drugs to speed labor, episiotomy, cesarean, etc.), she usually favors natural approaches to birth and is well equipped to _Assist_ the mother through the emotional journey without the use of these interventions.

I feel that every woman deserves the support and _Assistance_ of a doula at her birth.

Opportunity to Serve Our Sisters

As AMANI Birth rolls out, there will be more and more doulas available to serve women worldwide, _in sha' Allah_. Because of its _Islamic_ foundation, it will provide services for our _Muslimah_ sisters who may otherwise have to rely on non-_Muslims_ for support and guidance. While there is not necessarily anything wrong with this, there is certainly a benefit to trusting that your _Muslimah_ sister will have a better understanding of issues of religious modesty and customs that her counterpart would not.

If you are passionate about birth and feel a calling to help women during this time with education and/or labor support, I'd encourage you to consider becoming an AMANI-Birth Educator and Doula. In remembrance and obedience to what the Messenger of Allah (_sallallahu `alayhi wa sallam_) said,

"Whoever relieves his brother [or sister] of a hardship from the hardships of this world, Allah shall relieve him of a hardship from the hardships of the Day of Judgment. And whoever makes things easy for a person in difficulty, Allah will ease for him in this world and the Next. And whoever conceals (the faults of) a Muslim, Allah will conceal him in this world and the Next. Allah is forever aiding a slave so long as he is in the aid of his brother." [Sahih Muslim, al-Tirmidhi, Ibn Majah *and others*]

After all, what better way to relieve your sister of hardship than by <u>Assisting</u> her through the labor and birth of her child?

CHAPTER 6

What to Expect in <u>AMANI Birth</u> Training-Part One

<u>AMANI Birth</u> classes are perfect for expectant mothers who want the benefit of live instruction to help them prepare for their upcoming births. Some mothers take the classes alone, while others bring their husbands or other support persons along. Either way, it's a great place to meet other soon-to-be mothers while having access to <u>AMANI Birth</u> professionals who can guide you along the way, *in sha' Allah*.

The first section comes from the *Assisting* Series and focuses on "Being the Best Coach" for the pregnant and laboring mother. Regardless if you are her husband, mother, sister, friend, nurse, midwife, doctor, or professional labor companion (doula), it is important that you work with the woman in a way that will empower her to birth her baby with the least amount of intervention and interference possible. For some women that may mean simply being nearby in case she calls out to you and for others it may mean having a constant presence with lots of loving encouragement and physical support. It's our obligation to have intuition, patience, strength, stamina, and most important, respect for the woman in labor.

When a woman and her labor companion embark on <u>AMANI Birth</u> training they will explore a series of modules to help them understand the labor and birth process, to learn about the many options involved in birthing, and to sort out their priorities for birth. Upon doing so they will rehearse their birth experience through discussion and activity in order to formulate a birth plan that best communicates the birth experience they pray for.

In this way, both mother and her companion(s) will be on the same page and will be able to work together as a coherent team to achieve the best start in life for the baby and the family, *in sha' Allah*. Knowing what to expect and having a rehearsed plan of action, will serve to ease tension and fear, thereby reducing stress and unnecessary pain and discomfort for the mother, *in sha' Allah*. It will also help her companion to understand his/her role and provide the framework for him/her to advocate for the mother and baby during the labor and birth based on knowledge of the birth process as well as understanding of the mother's needs and preferences.

The *Assisting* series is compiled of four modules:

Module1   Mother's Needs in Pregnancy

We will explore the mother's needs so that her companion can help and encourage her in her preparation for the birth. It's important to understand that during pregnancy she is likely to experience a roller coaster of emotions and will need extra love and support. All through pregnancy, labor and birth there is a complex interaction of hormones at play.

Most pregnant woman are notably more needy, emotional, and anxious. The intensity of these needs and emotions grows in pace with her belly. The companion should be compassionate with regard to her increasing needs for love, encouragement, and support.

A good companion takes his/her role to protect and support her seriously and creates an environment of loving care where the expectant mother feels safe to relax and allow her emotional guard down. This is an important part of her preparation for birth so that she can explore her vulnerabilities and process her feelings of fear and anxiety about her imminent future, as well as deal with any past traumas or hurts that will inevitably come up during the intense emotional stages of labor and birth.

We will also briefly discover the special care to be given to diet and exercise during pregnancy. These factors are vitally important so that she can maintain her health and prepare herself physically for the hard work of birthing.

Labor is probably the most physically challenging event she will ever tackled and it is an injustice to her and her baby if approached without proper preparation. The companion's duty at this time is to learn her diet and exercise needs. He/she can then encourage her to meet her nutritional and physical goals.

Sometimes just knowing that someone else is looking into and caring for her eating and exercising habits is enough to keep her on track. At other times he/she may have to step in with loving involvement to support her in maintaining her healthy eating and exercise routine that will ensure she and her baby remain as low risk as possible for the best chance at a normal, natural birth.

Module 2   Mother's Needs in Labor and Birth

The mother's needs during labor and birth are similar to that of pregnancy. Except this will be the time that she will really need to employ all of the physical flexibility and stamina she prepared for during her pregnancy. Labor will likely challenge her beyond her expectations and she will need strong, encouraging companions to get her through. When she feels she's hit a wall, her companions must be prepared to push her that extra mile; they must believe in her ability to make it through in order to provide her the boost of strength that comes from loving support and encouragement during the toughest part of her journey.

Mentally she will need peace and tranquility to be able to tune into her body and allow herself to let go and surrender to the hard work of labor and birth. She needs a clear mind, free of stress and anxiety, so that she can relax and work with her body at this intense time. It is the duty of her labor companion(s) to set the mood and the pace. Everyone in attendance should be calming and supportive of the mother. If anyone present causes her tension or stress, they should leave the scene without making issue or hurt feelings. The mother's ability to find a mental place of serenity overrides anyone else's desire to attend the birth.

The importance of her emotional state cannot be underestimated. This equates to how she feels about her situation. This involves both her current life situation and how she feels about transitioning from pregnant woman to new mother, as well as how she feels at any given moment about her birthplace and the persons involved in her birth. Any unresolved feelings will likely creep up during the birth and could cause the mother anxiety and stress which can release hormones that can potentially interfere with the process of labor and render it more painful and ineffective.

Her companion should focus on providing a protected and loving environment for her to safely journey into the unknown. Birth is as intimate an event as the intercourse that got her here. She must feel secure to experience her vulnerability at this time in order to allow the rush of intense hormones to sweep over her and serve as the driving and guiding force during her labor and birth. Dr. Bradley made a statement in his book, _Husband-Coached Childbirth_, "**The loving encouragement from a trained coach can do more for the comfort and relaxation of his wife than any amount of medication.**" I agree but might reword it to say that the support, advocacy, and protection of her companion(s) will do more for her labor and birth than any synthetic drug or medical procedure.

Module 3   Birth Team Roles

Everyone at the birth has a role to play. However, only the mother can **give** birth. Of course, a skilled surgeon or birth attendant can intervene with a myriad of drugs, protocols, and procedures to **deliver** her of her burden, but with a hefty physical and emotional price to her and her baby. It's important that everyone involved know that this mother is not just handing her body over for **delivery**. But she is rather seeking loving support so that she can **give** birth to her baby naturally, in the most loving, gentle way possible, _in sha' Allah_.

In this regard, all persons involved should respect the mother's birth plans. These plans were made with careful consideration, knowledge of options, attention to priorities, and preparation to back them up. It is the mother's role to tap into her inner strength and resources and to carefully **listen** to her body's cues during labor and birth. Her intuition should be trusted and her needs met.

The labor companion, or coach, knows her well. He/she has been working with her during the pregnancy to prepare for the big event of birth. They have rehearsed the birth scene many times by now and he/she is well equipped to support and encourage her through even the roughest parts of labor. His/her role is that of loving and tender guide, giving her **permission** to surrender to her journey while ensuring she never travels alone. He/she is also her advocate and protector from the outside world as she delves far inside herself in focus and in search for the inner strength necessary to meet the challenges of the day.

If a professional doula is present, it usually relieves much stress on both the mother and her close companion(s). The doula's trusted experience and outer level of protection are priceless during the most intense moments of labor. Her role is to encourage both the mother and her companion and to provide reassurance during any moments of doubt. She also serves as a translator of medical terminology and a reminder of the mother's desire to stick to her birth plan. She is a calming force during any moments of storm. Although she cannot make decisions for the mother, she can gently remind her of the birth experience and carefully laid plan and help everyone remain focused on supporting the mother through it.

The birth attendant's (usually a doctor or midwife) role is that of patient and quiet observer. He/she should not interfere unless there is a true medical emergency. Routines and protocols have no place in a natural, well prepared for birth. Sometimes this is the hardest part of being an attendant at a natural birth. Trusting *Allah's* design for birth can be difficult when one has been taught to trust themselves, their tonics, and their scalpels even more. However, the birth attendant who understands their role as a lifeguard, and only gets wet if someone is drowning, is worth their weight in gold.

Module 4   Making the Birth Plan

During AMANI Birth classes, the woman and her companion(s) will explore her needs and their desires for their birth experience. They will formulate a birth plan assuming normality and based on knowledge and personal priorities. Within that context is the responsibility to exercise good birth consumerism in finding a birth team and a birthplace that trusts *Allah's* design for birth and that respects the woman's hard work in preparing to take advantage of the many safeguards of birth.

Along with this is the responsibility for decisions. Decisions about protocols, procedures, medications, positions, and a host of other factors should be left to the mother, unless an emergency arises. Once she has selected a birth team she trusts to support her in her choices, she needs to let go and keep the lines of communication, and her mind, open so that she can remain respectful and flexible, should her birth become complicated and a need for intervention arise.

One thing is certain, her birth will not go according to plan if she hasn't taken the time to research, prepare, and make one. This is an important part of the preparation process and should be taken seriously. Likewise, it should be respected as an important blueprint for her labor and all persons involved with her birth should have the consideration to read it, become familiar with it, and support it to the best of their abilities.

PART TWO - *MOTHERS*

With *Motherhood* comes *Allah's* command for honor and respect from our children. But this comes with a price. For it is *Mothers* alone who bear the burden of pregnancy and pains of childbirth and upon her is the child's dependence for two years.

> **"And [God says:] 'We have enjoined upon man goodness towards his parents: his *Mother* bore him by bearing strain upon strain, and his utter dependence on her lasted two years: [hence, O man,] be grateful towards Me and towards thy parents, [and remember that] with Me is all journeys' end.** [Qur'an 31:14]

What is birth if not all about *Mothers*? AMANI Birth was born out of our desire to support and educate *Mothers*, their birth companions, and the birthing community about the inherent safeties built into *Allah's* perfect design for birth. With this comes the *Mother's* responsibility to prepare for her birth and her partner's obligation to assist her in doing so.

As a *Mother* myself, I know the joy and triumph of birthing my children naturally. *Alhamdulillah*, I know the blessings and rewards of feeling great after bringing my children into the world by trusting the Creator's design of my body to do so; without succumbing to the myriad of interventions pushed on us in the hospital birth setting. I also know the preparation, determination, strength, confidence, and trust it takes to do so amidst the challenges of today's medical model of birth.

AMANI Birth is for *Mothers*, about *Mothers*, and for the loving people who support them in birth. But, it is also about babies. We mustn't lose touch with the fact that this is the baby's birth. It's so important to understand that whatever the baby experiences will affect him/her lifelong and will play a part in developing their sense of trust and self-confidence. The birth experience effects how we react to the world around us—lifelong.

CHAPTER 7

Who is <u>AMANI Birth</u> for?

<u>AMANI Birth</u> is for any woman who seeks the best birth experience for herself and her baby and who is willing to work for it. <u>AMANI Birth</u> <u>*Mothers*</u> increase their knowledge of the natural birth process and demand respect and choices in their birth. They devote their pregnancy to eating healthy, exercising, and to preparing themselves physically, mentally, and emotionally for their pending births.

When it comes to navigating the medical model of birth, knowledge really is power. The more you understand how your body works in labor, the less likely you are to fight the natural process inadvertently. In addition, you will learn how to actually work <u>with</u> your body to get the most of its natural power and instinct.

Dr. Sarah Buckley eloquently addresses the medical profession in her book, *Gentle Birth, Gentle Mothering*, as she explains that women should feel confident to use the medical support system as a safety net, without becoming entangled by submitting to it. This truly is at the heart of the vision for <u>AMANI Birth</u> as a childbirth education and birth attendant training and certification program.

Protecting *Mothers* and Babies

It takes both sides of the field, _Mothers_ and their close companion(s), together with the professional birth team, to protect the birth experience for the _Mother_ and her baby in a gentle and safe way. Birth should never be a trauma and everyone needs to work together to ensure that the integrity, respect, and worship of *Allah*, the Designer and Creator, are not left out of the process by lack of trust in HIS infinite wisdom.

It's safe to say that _Mothers_ are naturally protective of their babies. AMANI Birth focuses not only on providing a natural birth experience for _Mother_ but also on a gentle beginning for baby, *in sha' Allah*. There can really be no compromise on either side, yet there must be sacrifice on the part of the _Mother_ to remain strong and steadfast during her labor and birth, if not for her own best experience, then for that of her baby.

Sacrifice for Baby's Sake

In fact, the _Mother's_ never-ending, selfless sacrifice for her child begins at the moment of conception and grows in immense measure, alongside her baby. Her unwavering duty to put her child first and to carry on in her journey of _Motherhood_ is a fitting reason for *Allah's* command to honor and respect her first and foremost, even three times more than that of the father.

> *The Prophet Muhammad said, may Allah's peace and blessings be upon him: Your Heaven lies under the feet of your mother.* (Ahmad, Nasai).

> *A man came to the Prophet and said, 'O Messenger of God! Who among the people is the most worthy of my good companionship? The Prophet said: Your* Mother. *The man said, 'Then who?' The Prophet said: Then your* Mother. *The man further asked, 'Then who?' The Prophet said: Then your* Mother. *The man asked again, 'Then who?' The Prophet said: Then your father.* (Bukhari, Muslim)

CHAPTER 8

Physiology of Pregnancy

When considering the physiology of pregnancy, it is difficult not to feel in awe of the Creator.

O MEN! If you are in doubt as to the [truth of] resurrection, [remember that,] verily, We have created [every one of] you out of dust, then out of a drop of sperm, then out of a germ-cell, then out of an embryonic lump complete [in itself] and yet incomplete so that We might make [your origin] clear unto you. And whatever We will [to be born] We cause to rest in the [Mothers'] wombs for a term set [by Us], and then We bring you forth as infants and [allow you to live] so that [some of] you might attain to maturity: for among you are such as are caused to die [in childhood], just as many a one of you is reduced in old age to a most abject state, ceasing to know anything of what he once knew so well. And [if, O man, thou art still in doubt as to resurrection, consider this:] thou canst see the earth dry and lifeless - and [suddenly,] when We send down waters upon it, it stirs and swells and puts forth every kind of lovely plant! [Qur'an 22:5]

In the preceding verse, the divinity of *Allah* is so clearly described in relation to the amazing scientific discoveries we have since made. The modern, worldly evidence provides support for what we were already informed by our Creator so many years ago. Truly, these are proofs for those who think, *subhan'Allah!*

Another amazing proof is the stages of gestation taking place within the protection of the mother's abdomen, womb, and the placenta. Modern medicine has divided our pregnancy into three unique parts or trimesters. But long before there was medical study, there was the *Qur'an*.

> *He has created you [all] out of one living entity, and out of it fashioned its mate; and he has bestowed upon you four kinds of cattle of either sex; [and] He creates you in your* <u>*Mothers'*</u> *wombs,* <u>*one act of creation after another, in threefold depths of dark-*</u><u>*ness.*</u> *Thus is God, your Sustainer: unto Him belongs all dominion: there is no deity save Him: how, then, can you lose sight of the truth?* [Qur'an30:6]

Allah's Creation

Pregnancy is one of the most amazing times in a woman's life. It is humbling to serve a role in the design of a new human being. As we watch our bellies grow and feel our babies' movements we bear witness to the incredible creation, so perfectly orchestrated, as it unfolds within our own bodies. Most women also recognize the honor and blessing of carrying this great responsibility. Being part of this grand miracle is a reminder for thankfulness.

> *It is HE who has created you [all] out of one living entity, and out of it brought into being its mate, so that man might incline [with love] towards woman. And so, when he has embraced her, she conceives [what at first is] a light burden, and continues to bear it. Then, when she grows heavy [with child], they both call unto God, their Sustainer, "If Thou indeed grant us a sound [child], we shall most certainly be among the grateful!"* [Qur'an 7:189]

Allah has provided a series of complex systems that carefully work together from conception to birth. Pregnancy is one of the safest times in our lives, *alhamdulillah*. The baby is enveloped in these systems, which protect the baby during pregnancy labor and birth.

Baby's Physiological Protection

The baby has his/her own bones, which transform and go through stages of flexible cartilage to strong supportive bone mass. The muscles and skin also serve as protection as does the thick white cream (called vernix caseosa), which coats the skin to protect from the watery environment of the womb. The water (called amniotic fluid) is constantly being manufactured by the *Mother's* body and protects the baby from infection and by equalizing pressure and regulating temperature. Like a ball inside a water balloon, it would take a very severe blow to the *Mother's* stomach to injure the baby.

Mother's Physiological Protection

The *Mother's* body also serves as a source of nourishment and protection for the baby. The womb itself is a strong band of muscles that encase and protect the baby. They also work with amazing precision and force during labor and birth to efficiently expel the baby at the end of the pregnancy term. The pelvis forms a hard cradle of support for the baby as well. The outer muscles, fat, and skin also wrap the baby in a warm and protected environment during pregnancy. Enough cannot be said of the Kegel muscle (pelvic floor) and its role in supporting all of the *Mother's* internal organs in addition to the baby. A tone, firm Kegel will ensure the easiest delivery of the baby as he/she passes through this muscle to be born, *in sha' Allah*. (See Chapter 14 for details about the Kegel muscles and exercises.)

Physiological Perspective

Obviously, the expectant *Mother* can expect to experience a myriad of changes as her body evolves to support the life of her child. These changes can be uncomfortable at times, but when they are viewed as the amazing signs from *Allah* and proof of the mastery of HIS design, they are thrilling and rewarding signs of the direct result of divinity through us.

Pregnancy is an honor and a blessing and is a time of extreme trust: Trust **of** *Allah* in our ability to bear the burden, and Trust **in** *Allah* not to burden us with more than we can bear. In fact, there are at least four *ayats* (verses) in *Qur'an* about our burdens:

> **"God does not burden any soul with more than he is well able to bear..."** [Qur'an 2:286]
>
> **"... We do not burden any soul with more than he is well able to bear......"** [Qur'an 6:152]
>
> **"...We do not burden any soul with more than he is well able to bear..."** [Qur'an 7:42]
>
> **"...God does not burden any human being with more than He has given him - [and it may well be that] God will grant, after hardship, ease.** [Qur'an 65:7]

It's important to understand that the changes our bodies go through provide nourishment and protection for our babies as well as safeguard our own lives for the birthing event. When we take the time to learn about these physiological changes, it becomes apparent what miracles they truly are. With this mindset, it becomes much easier to enjoy pregnancy and make the minor sacrifices needed to take the best care of ourselves, for our baby's sake and our own, at this time.

How we experience life really boils down to our perspective and trust in *Allah's* perfect plan for us. If we can view pregnancy, labor, and birth as normal, positive events in our life, they most likely will be. However, if we view them as an illness, hardship, hassle, or pain, they likely will be. This also holds true for those around us during this time. Surrounding ourselves with positive, empowering people will make a difference in our experience, *in sha' Allah*. This is especially important during the vulnerable peak of labor and birth.

Safeguards and Sacrifices

A few examples to think about, when considering automatic changes during pregnancy, are the increased blood volume and the expansion of joints. These are both causes for complaint, until we look at the amazing safeguards they provide at birth.

First of all, the pregnant woman's digestion and blood circulation slow down during pregnancy so that it can absorb more of the nutrients from her food in order to support the growing baby. Of course, these slowed processes can cause fatigue and nausea, especially in the first months. However, by the second trimester, she will begin to gain more blood volume, *in sha' Allah*, which will serve to relieve her fatigue.

In fact, her blood volume typically increases by about fifty percent during pregnancy. This can cause complaints of bleeding gums or frequent nose bleeds. However, this is truly amazing when we look at the inevitability of blood loss at birth, *subhan'Allah*.

Allah (SWT) has built-in this safety net to give the Mother allowance to bleed at birth, Allahu Akbar! The <u>Mother</u> must focus her attention on her nutrition in order to support this normal increase of blood volume. It is very important that she has an adequate intake of iron and water, and that she continues to salt her food to taste. As Anne Frye mentions in her book, <u>Holistic Midwifery, A Comprehensive Textbook for Midwives in Homebirth Practice, Volume I, Care During Pregnancy</u>, salt is necessary for proper expansion of blood volume. Dr. Tomas Brewer also made this point in his prenatal nutrition classes as well.

Protein is another major factor in growing a new person from scratch, after all, every cell in our body is essentially made up of protein. Not only that, having at least 75 grams of protein daily has been shown to reduce the risk of metabolic toxemia of late pregnancy, one of the common diseases of pregnancy that can result in maternal convulsions, premature birth, and even death for <u>Mother</u> and child. It's vitally important that <u>Mothers</u> *pay close attention to what foods they choose so that they can get the most out of each bite.*

This can be a challenge for <u>Mothers</u> who are accustomed to eating at whim, especially if their diets are typically full of carbohydrates, sweets, and sodas and void of water, milk, fresh fruits, vegetables, and proteins. But the sacrifice becomes easier when we realize the importance diet plays in the natural increase of blood volume, which we need to be at its peak for birth, growth of our baby, and the health of *Mother* and child, *in sha' Allah*.

As for the joints, there are hormones at play during the pregnancy that work to loosen joints and soften cartilage. This loosening affects all the *Mother's* joints and can bring complaints of wobbliness in the hips or clumsiness in the fingers. Some *Mothers* even experience mild pains in wrists and other joints. However, this is an extremely important part of the body's preparation for birth. It allows the *Mother's* pelvis to expand in order to accommodate the baby passing through it. Of course, no one enjoys the added clumsiness or discomfort during pregnancy; however, understanding where it comes from, and why it is so important, helps *Mothers* to view it as the miracle it is, rather than dwell on the discomforts of it.

Listen to Your Body

Our body also gives us signs to help us modify our behavior for the safety of our baby. For example, the nausea and vomiting, often associated with pregnancy, can be caused by low blood sugar or poor nutrition. This is a sign for *Mother* to slow down, eat well, and rest often.

But this is just one small example of the many signals our bodies' send us during pregnancy. In fact, a *Mother's* instincts are strong with regard to her pregnancy, labor, birth, baby, and beyond, *masha'Allah*. Unfortunately, we have been blasted with media and medical messages that may leave us in self-doubt, or worse, repressing the instincts, which are there to guide and protect us.

Often times, it takes a very traumatic experience for parents to snap out of the virtual coma induced by outside influence and advice. In fact, I find that the healing take-away from an emotionally or physically challenging birth experience can be an epiphany for parents who are then able to reach deep within themselves to realize that they truly know what's best for themselves and their family. Pregnancy, labor, and birth often serve as a training ground for parenting. Once we learn to tune into ourselves and trust the signals of our body, we have taken a monumental step towards trusting our instincts and parenting our child lifelong, *in sha' Allah.*

Danger Signs to Report

It is important that the <u>Mother</u> is aware of danger signs during pregnancy and report them immediately to her medical care provider. This includes:

1. Abdominal pain, especially sudden, sharp, continuing pain.

2. Vaginal bleeding.

3. Persistent vomiting, especially past the first trimester.

4. Illness and/or high fever.

5. Painful urination or difficulty urinating (may be urinary tract infection, which can lead to preterm labor and birth, do not ignore this).

6. Unusual vaginal discharge, itching, burning, or "fishy" odor.

7. Sudden decrease or absence of baby's movements.

8. Dizziness, especially persistent or with headache or visual disturbances.

9. Excessive swelling (some swelling is normal, especially in the legs and feet after a long day on your feet or seated at a desk or in a car for prolonged periods), especially in the face and/or upper extremities.

10. Sudden gush of water from the vagina.

11. Anything coming out of the vagina, such as the bag of waters, umbilical cord, hand, foot, etc.

Rest assured that pregnancy is typically a very healthy time, especially when the woman eats well and stays active. Just be aware of your body, seek appropriate prenatal care, and listen to your intuition.

CHAPTER 9

Physiology of Labor and Birth

Labor is an intense, yet amazing process of transformation from pregnant woman to _Mother_. It is the climax of a journey and will likely be remembered in great detail for decades to come, _masha'Allah_. Understanding the process and knowing what to expect before traveling through it can make the difference between a triumphant or traumatizing birth experience, _in sha' Allah_.

In fact, thinking of labor like a journey reminds me of one of the many _duas_ (supplications) for traveling: "**O Allah, make our journey easy and roll up its distance. O Allah, you are the companion on the journey and the successor over the family. O Allah, protect me from the toils of the journey, miserable sights and ill fated outcome with wealth and family.**" [_Muslim_]

What a nice prayer for the journey to _Motherhood_! It's a good reminder that _Allah_ has the power to make it short and we should turn to HIM for protection and best outcomes.

Importance of the Birth Experience

Enough cannot be said about the importance of this experience for the _Mother_, baby, family and society at large. How a woman and baby experience their birth together can set the stage for their bonding and the _Mother_/child relationship lifelong. It will also make a lasting imprint on the baby's psyche and will impact how he/she relates to and trusts the world around him/her.

It's also important to consider that birth can either be an empowering high for the _Mother_ or a depressing emotional trauma. In fact, it's well known that _Mothers_ who experience highly medical births are more prone to postpartum depression and some are even diagnosed with Post Traumatic Stress Disorder as a result.

In fact, one well-resourced study about post-traumatic stress disorder in new mothers stated **"Women who developed PTSD symptoms had a higher prevalence of 'traumatic' previous childbirth, with subsequent depression and anxiety. They also reported more medical complications..."** I think it's fair to say that every woman longs for a birth experience to celebrate, rather than heal from, whether that healing be physical or emotional!

Know What to Expect

When I think of any long journey I have taken, it's always amazing to me to note that the return trip typically seems shorter than the initial travel. I believe this is due, in part, to the familiarity of having been on this road before. Somehow, knowing what to expect makes even the most grueling journey more bearable.

Having worked for years with the American Automobile Association in the States, I recall the many travelers who came in for road maps and tour books before embarking on long trips. Couple this familiarity with preparation, and the journey often becomes as exciting as the actual destination. In fact, it is often said that it's not only the destination that matters, but equally as much, it's the journey. I also often find that there is a second wind or burst of energy, as any long journey (including labor) comes to an end.

This view that knowing what to expect makes things easier is a stark difference from some medical professionals who feel that the patient is better off not knowing what to expect. I suppose that may be true in surgeries and complicated medical procedures. But when we view birth as a normal life event to be supported and celebrated, why are we hiding the information that will serve the woman well in learning to work with her body?

I suppose it comes down to a matter of perception and roles. If you see birth as medical procedure with the doctor or other care provider as the one in charge and the patient as ignorant and submissive to delivery, then I suppose the "you don't need to know" attitude might fit. However, you see birth as a natural life event with the doctor or other care provider as a guide and lifeguard who watches over a woman giving birth, whose role it is to support her on her journey, rather than taking it over, then knowledge is the power she needs to prepare.

Stages of Labor

Labor is divided into three stages. During the first stage the womb is working hard to open in preparation for the actual birth. Second stage refers to the actual birth; at this time the _Mother_ works with her womb to push the baby out. Third stage occurs after the birth and refers to the expulsion of the placenta.

Understanding how the body functions, allows women to maximize the natural event and work with, rather than against, their bodies. In doing so, the birth becomes easier and unnecessary pain can be avoided, _in sha'Allah_. Additionally, understanding the process alleviates fear and tension, which can interfere with labor and cause increased pain.

On my Saudi Life Motherhood column, I wrote an article, "Waiting for Labor". In this article, I describe the stages of labor:

Waiting for Labor

ANYONE partaking in labor and birth would agree that they are amazing events to behold. They are also probably the most intense moments of a woman's life. The final journey from pregnant woman to _Mother_ can be overwhelming in its uncertain mysteries and infinite variations.

While waiting for labor, it benefits couples to learn what to expect. Having an understanding of the process can help a woman cope during this vulnerable and sometimes frightening time. Fortunately, we have come a long way in the study of the birth process and can divide it into three distinct stages.

First Stage Labor

The first stage of labor is the period of time when the contractions of the uterus begin until it's time to push the baby out the birth canal. The contractions in this stage usually start out mild and gradually build in intensity and frequency. First stage labor is further divided into three parts:

1. Early First Stage – Usually characterized by mild, squeezing contractions

2. Active First Stage – Typically stronger, more intense, hardening contractions

3. Transition – Contractions change to expulsive in nature

During first stage labor many things are occurring to prepare the _Mother_ and baby for birth. Amazingly her body works by itself at this time and _Mother's_ job is simply to **relax and let it happen**. The most measurable event is the uterus (womb) opening in preparation to deliver the baby (dilation of the cervix).

Transition is typically the shortest, but often the most difficult part of the entire labor. It is a time of major change in the way the labor feels which can bring confusion, self-doubt and panic for the unsuspecting _Mother_. This is often the time that women ask for medicinal pain relief, cry, or feel they simply can't go on. The good news is that all of these emotions are normal signs of progression and usually indicate that the pushing stage isn't too far off. Expecting and recognizing the emotional signs of transition make it much easier to manage through it.

Second Stage Labor

The second stage of labor is much different than the first. When a woman reaches this point, it's time for her to work with her body to push her baby out. It can be physically strenuous and exhausting, but it's also the most exhilarating as it ends with the birth of the baby.

Third Stage Labor

In the shadow of joyful emotions from the birth of the baby, this stage is almost ignored by most women. It is simply the part of labor when the placenta detaches from the uterine wall and is expelled. Most _Mothers_ are happily nursing and cuddling with their new baby and rarely even notice the momentary interruption.

Knowing and understanding the stages of labor can help to take some of the "mystery" out of birthing. I truly believe that women who attend antenatal classes and carefully prepare (physically, mentally, and emotionally) for their births will find it the most rewarding experience of their lives. Look to future articles for advice as to what to do/not do during labor as well as the physical and emotional characteristics of each stage, _insha'Allah_.

Emotional Behaviors in Labor

As important as it is to understand the physical stages of labor, it may be even more important to become familiar with emotions and behaviors that are common to each stage. There is a fairly predictable pattern to women's behaviors as they progress in their labors. It is especially important for labor companions to tune into the _Mother_ in order to best fulfill her needs.

On my Saudi Life Motherhood column, I wrote an article, "Coaching the Emotional Stages of Labor". In this article, I addressed labor coaches with information about recognizing the emotional needs of _Mothers_ at the various stages of labor:

Coaching the Emotional Stages of Labor

EVERY labor is different and each woman passes through it in her own way and at her own speed. Medical staff are trained to physically examine the woman throughout this time to try and assess her progress. The most notable measure is the opening of the womb, which typically dilates to an estimated 10 cm for birth.

However, there are many immeasurable events happening during this time as well. Sometimes doctors can get nervous if "measurable" progress isn't made according to some "normal" timetable. These immeasurables can include:

- Physical alignment of the baby to her pelvis
- Softening of her cartilages to allow the pelvis to expand
- Balancing of her hormones
- Production of immunities in her breast milk
- Various emotional stages as the woman transitions from pregnant woman to _Mother_

In fact a woman's emotional signs are often more indicative of which stage of labor she is in, than any physical exam given by her birth attendant. By noting her behaviors, a labor coach can not only gauge her progress, but also adjust his or her activities to best support her throughout this time.

Emotional Signs and Needs

Early First Stage

At the onset of labor, she may not be sure if it's really labor. She may seem excited or nervous as she begins to notice contractions. Some women become very restless and talkative. She will probably continue her regular daily routine. Often times she will be hungry at this time.

As a coach, it's important not to get too excited. This may or may not be true labor. It's best to encourage her to take a walk, eat, drink, shower, and then rest. Relax, you will know soon enough if it's true labor or not.

Established First Stage

As her labor becomes more established, she will realize, "This is it!" This acceptance may be exciting or overwhelming to her. She may need to stop what she's doing and concentrate during contractions. She may still be restless and talkative between contractions. She'll be mindful of the many changes taking place in her body.

The coach should encourage her to walk. Walking will open the inlet of the pelvis and is estimated to shorten labor by nearly 28% [although there needs to be more research done to substantiate this number]. The mother should have freedom of movement and the coach should be committed to staying with her from this point on. Timing contractions (from the start of one to the start of the next) can help to determine her labor rhythm.

Active/Late First Stage

As the labor intensifies, she will become serious and determined. She will seem to be working hard and may not want to be disturbed during contractions. She may begin to lose her modesty at this point. She may need to lie down and rest during contractions. She will most likely lose her appetite by this time. She may feel she needs the bathroom often.

It's very important that the coach keeps her environment peaceful and calm. Dim lights and quiet are what's usually needed now. She should be encouraged to drink and use the restroom often. This stage of labor can be hard work and she will really need emotional support and praise.

Transition

As her body transitions from first to second stage labor, she may become confused. It's common for women to be emotionally insecure during this phase. Many women will cry and feel overwhelmed. She may become frightened or want to give up. These are good signs and indicate that the baby is coming soon!

Recognizing transition is the most important thing a coach can do. She will need a lot of reassurance and encouragement now. She should not be disturbed. Remind her to take one contraction at a time. This is often the time women will ask for pain relief. You can help her to avoid drugs by reminding her that the hardest part is almost over. Although transition can be the most challenging part of labor, it usually doesn't last long (ten to thirty minutes). Tell her, she's doing great and assure her that she can do this!

Second Stage

This is the time for pushing the baby out. She will no longer be modest. She will gradually or suddenly feel an urge to push. She usually will get a burst of energy and become calm and determined to get it over with.

She will need a lot of loving encouragement and emotional support. If she has avoided pain medication she should have freedom of movement to choose the best position for her. Flat on her back, in stirrups may be the best position for doctors, but it's the absolute worst for her and her baby. The coach should remind her to completely relax between contractions to recoup her energy. Assuming she has not been placed on medication to rush her labor, she will usually enjoy longer rest periods between contractions. It's important that she take advantage of this gift of time from *Allah*. An unmedicated _Mother_ should be allowed to tune-in to her body and push to the point of comfort. Guided or directed pushing is best left for the medicated moms who cannot feel the contractions and natural cues of her body.

Third Stage

This is the easiest of all. This is simply the expulsion of the placenta after the birth of the baby. Most likely the _Mother_ is too excited and caught up in the relief and joy of birth to even notice.

It's paramount that baby be placed skin-to-skin with _Mother_ and be encouraged to nurse right away. The stimulation of baby's feeding will cause important uterine contractions that help expel the placenta, shrink the uterus, and prevent excessive maternal bleeding. The first few moments are sacred and mom, baby, and coach should be encouraged to gently and lovingly interact and bond with their new baby. Assuming the _Mother_ has had an unmedicated birth, there should be no reason to rush to clamp and cut the cord. I will highly recommend any doctor who recognizes the importance of these first moments by delaying cord clamping and not rushing to wash, weigh, or handle the baby.

This overview of the emotional stages of labor is a small sample from the Bradley Method® Student Workbook. When expectant _Mothers_ and their coaches are prepared for labor they usually find it easier and more enjoyable to birth their babies naturally, _in sha'Allah. Du'a_ for all our labors to be easy and our babies to be healthy and pleasing to _Allah_ and their parents... _AMEEN!_

Freedom of Movement

I cannot stress enough the importance of remaining active in labor for as long as possible. Freedom of movement is imperative and is proven to shorten labor. In fact, according to a Chocrane Library review of twenty-one studies, involving over 3,500 women, they found that, "**There is evidence that walking and upright positions in the first stage of labour reduce the length of labour and do not seem to be associated with increased intervention or negative effects on _Mothers'_ and babies' wellbeing. Women should be encouraged to take up whatever position they find most comfortable in the first stage of labour.**"]

CHAPTER 10

Enjoying the Birth Experience

Labor truly is hard work! Beyond being physically taxing, it can be emotionally draining as well as embarrassing. But take heart in knowing that it can be satisfying and empowering as well. Unfortunately, social inhibitions and embarrassment can often get in the way of experiencing the joys of birth. This is especially true for women with a high degree of modesty, such as most *Muslim* sisters (especially Arabs or others from Eastern cultures). It may well be the most vulnerable time for a woman; how she feels about her body, coupled with the treatment she receives by her caregivers, will make a world of difference in how she perceives the experience.

Birth is a Sexual Function

In consideration of simple anatomy, birth is an event of the sexual organs. You really cannot separate sexuality from birth. Pregnancy begins with the intimate sexual act and ends with the most exposed sexual performance of a woman's lifetime. To be on display, observed while clinically poked and prodded, goes against our natural need for privacy and intimacy when engaged in anything sexual.

Moreover, the hormones that a woman's body produces for birthing are the same hormones invoked in deep sexual encounters. Birthing in a strange environment (the hospital), with strangers watching (doctors and/or nurses), while being commanded about behaviors (including positions to take and noises to hush) is likely to make a woman feel extremely dominated and vulnerable.

Conversely, _Mothers_, who are free to be surrounded by people they love and trust, feel supported and are more likely to "let go" physically and emotionally and surrender to the instincts of birthing. When they are able to so, they are able to truly enjoy the birth experience.

However, we must also take into account the many drugs that may be offered or given (with or without consent), to speed the process or take away the sensations and feelings, which make the experience a far cry from the natural life-event that it truly is. Couple this with invasive medical procedures (needle insertions, fetal monitors strapped to the abdomen, incision in the genital area, possible surgical delivery, etc.) and it's understandable that most women do not see birth as an "enjoyable" experience, regardless of who is present with them. In fact, too many women suffer from some form or another of postpartum depression (as noted in the referenced research article in the previous chapter) due to emotional and/or physical trauma experienced in birth.

Healing From Birth

From my perspective, it is heartbreaking when the birth experience becomes an event to heal from, especially emotionally. When this happens, some _Mothers_ become fearful of becoming pregnant again. In fact, it is often times during their second or subsequent pregnancy that they begin to do their homework, research their options, and prepare themselves for the next birth. This is why many AMANI Birth students are veterans, having two or more children already.

By finding AMANI Birth, you have taken a first step towards this preparation, _masha'Allah_. For yours and your baby's sake, I hope this is your first birth, but even if not, I am very happy for you to be here amongst the pages of this book. If you are here because of prior birth trauma, I'd like to make *dua* for you that *Allah* grant you peace and reward you with ease for your time and effort to prepare for your next birth. Please take to heart that *Allah* promises that after every hardship comes ease.

"And, behold, with every hardship comes ease:verily, with every hardship comes ease!" *[Qur'an 94:5-6]*

Joyful Birth

The good news is that birth doesn't have to be a trauma! It can be a truly empowering event to joyfully remember for a lifetime, *in sha'Allah*. In part this is dependent upon the caregiver who assists in your birth. It's important you find someone who is a "caregiver, whose purpose it is to assist," rather than the more common, "healthcare provider who dominates." Building rapport and a trusting relationship with your caregiver should be one of the priorities of your prenatal care, *in sha'Allah*.

When women realize that only they can birth their babies and take responsibility to do so, the experience becomes empowering. Rather than turning her body over to the unknown mystery of birth and fearfully trusting strangers to get her through it, she learns how the body functions during labor and birth and prepares herself to work with her body to minimize the pain and discomfort experienced. It also helps to know that the majority of labor discomfort ends the second the baby is born, assuming she birthed without medical intervention and medications.

The intensity of the birth is quickly replaced with the intensity of bonding with the new baby. This is very different than a medical birth where the pain begins when the drugs wear off and the <u>Mother</u> spends the first precious moments (days, weeks, and even months) recovering from her birth trauma, which can greatly interfere in bonding with her precious newborn.

Trust *Allah*

Keep in mind that *Allah* created your body to birth; HIS design is not faulty. It is a rare few who truly need medical intervention, especially if they have taken the time to prepare and have worked hard to stay healthy and low-risk. Don't make the mistake of trading a day of labor for days of recovery. The time, effort, and determination put in before and during the labor pay off when it counts most, when your baby is in your arms, *in sha'Allah*.

Choosing Your Birth Attendant

Ideally, your birth attendant should be trained in the natural process of birth, recognizing problems, managing them naturally whenever possible, and resorting to medical intervention only when truly necessary. If your birth attendant is not supportive of truly natural birth, virtually untimed, unrushed, undrugged, and un-interfered, I urge you to shop around. Keep looking until you find the gem in your community. Finding a supportive, skilled attendant is half the battle; preparing yourself for the event is the other.

It is our sincerest desire for you to enjoy the kind of birth experience that leaves you soaring with self-confidence, empowered, and eager to _Mother_ the new life that has entered your world, *in sha' Allah*.

CHAPTER 11

Postpartum Recovery

Regardless of how good your birth experience is, <u>all</u> <u>*Mothers*</u> need recovery. After the birth, the womb will have an open site where the placenta was once attached. There should be no pain from this site, but it is a source of bleeding. The uterine muscles, however, may be sore, as you would expect any muscle group to be after a good strong workout.

After Pains

Allah (SWT) has built in important safety features for the postpartum process. One is the natural contraction of the uterus as the baby nurses. These contractions, sometimes called "after pains," may cause some discomfort, but it's far less than the pain of labor, *alhamdulillah*. They serve an important role in shrinking the uterus and clamping down the open blood vessels at the placental site. This works to minimize blood loss for the <u>*Mother*</u>.

Another feature of the natural process is the increased blood supply that the <u>*Mother*</u> should have experienced during her pregnancy, assuming she maintained a balanced diet, complete with adequate water intake and normal use of salt. This added blood volume will allow her to experience blood loss without endangering her life, *in sha' Allah*. Of course, her care provider will likely monitor her to ensure that she is within the normal range and she should report bleeding that seems extremely heavy during her postpartum period. In fact, soaking more than one large size feminine pad an hour is too much and her bleeding should substantially decrease by the second or third day.

It's important that the _Mother's_ diet continue to be balanced in order to support her healing and to provide for the needs of her nursing infant, _insha'Allah_. Vitamins A and C foods are especially important during this time as they facilitate healing. As noted above, breastfeeding is an important part of the process for the _Mother's_ healing as much as it is for the baby's nourishment.

Moreover, the first excretions from the breast, called colostrum, come as a yellowish, thick and sticky substance, often referred to as "liquid gold." This valuable "milk" is short on _quantity_ but just the right amount for the newborn's tiny stomach, which is literally the size of a pea at birth. Don't let anyone tell you that your first milk is no good or not enough or that your baby needs formula until your "real" milk comes in. Giving formula bottles because of these myths will only serve to disrupt your breastfeeding relationship and overextend your baby's stomach.

In fact, I'm always disturbed when _Mothers_ who want to exclusively breastfeed, are told by medical professionals (be they doctors, midwives, nurses, or hospital lactation consultants) that they MUST supplement with formula until the real milk comes in. I really have to wonder where they get their training with regard to breastfeeding, or if they truly have any at all.

Enough cannot be said about the value and _quality_ of colostrum (the first milk). It acts as a laxative to rid the newborn intestine of the first, thick, sticky bowel movements, called meconium, as well as lining the gut with healthy flora while providing important antibodies to the baby. None of this is possible if the baby is fed manmade formula instead.

Pain "Down There"

Depending on whether the perineal tissues (area between the vagina and anus) were compromised or not, she may experienced localized pain in this region, as well as need time to heal. Listed below are some tips for dealing with this discomfort:

1. Be sure you have a blow up swim ring to sit on so that you are not putting pressure on the sore area.

2. Use clean water (preferably distilled) in a squirt bottle to rinse the area after using the toilet. It's best not to use the bidet or water sprayer of the house as there may be many microorganisms in the typical home water supply.

3. Pat dry with toilet paper, never rub.

4. Avoid washing with soap.

5. Lightly dampen a feminine pad with clean water (preferably distilled) and keep it in the freezer. This way, when you change your pad after toileting, you can apply the cool pad for relief of pain.

6. Consider sleeping bare, in order for air to circulate the area, with an absorbent pad under you to protect the bed.

7. In Robin Lim's book, <u>After the Baby's Birth</u>, she advises sun bathing the affected tissues, as direct sunlight will warm the area and promotes faster healing. Of course, you'd need a private area that is exposed to sun in order to do so. She also says not to expose the area to sunlight if you are suffering a herpes outbreak, as the herpes virus thrives on ultraviolet light.

8. Keep your legs close together so as not to tug on stitches, if you have any.

9. Do Kegel exercises as soon as possible to pull tissues together and bring blood to the area for faster healing (See Chapter 14).

10. Sit in a shallow water (sitz) bath to soak the area.

Although perineal trauma can be quite painful, it usually heals well within six weeks. Possibly more importantly is learning how to prevent tears and cuts in the first place!

Avoiding the "Cut"

If the _Mother_ prepared her body nutritionally and physically and learned about self-directed, controlled pushing, chances are good she will have no cuts or tears, need no stitches, and feel little to no pain in this area, _in sha'Allah._

A well-prepared _Mother_ with a supportive birth attendant should not "need" an episiotomy (cut in the perineum to medically widen the vagina for birth). In fact, one question I would ask a potential care provide is their episiotomy rates and more importantly, their feelings with regards to the "necessity" of episiotomies, especially for first time _Mothers_. If the doctor seems leery of foregoing the cut or says that the majority of first time _Mothers_ "need" episiotomy, I'd personally run in the opposite direction! To me this indicates that the doctor is not assessing the woman's tissues, control of her pushing, or anything else about her as an individual and is treating birth as a routine, rather than the unique event that it is for each woman.

If the doctor is concerned about a stitching up a jagged tear versus a straight cut, I'd be leery of their suturing skills. What you need to realize is that the reason a tear is jagged is that tears occur in the liquid spaces between cells, the individual cells themselves are not compromised, whereas scissors cut through individual cells. Therefore, making a deliberate cut is more painful and more difficult to heal than a natural tear. Not to mention the fact that a cut **must** be sutured whereas a tear may not occur at all or be so minor that it doesn't need stitching.

On my Saudi Life Motherhood column, I wrote an article, "Many Mothers Routinely Cut at Delivery". In this article, I addressed the barbaric routine of cutting the _Mother's_ tissues in order to enlarge the vaginal opening for birth. You may want to read the comments online that followed this article:

Many _Mothers_ Routinely "Cut" at Delivery

THERE is a dreaded procedure routinely performed on expectant _Mothers_ that makes most cringe and fear their birth experience. It's called an episiotomy. An episiotomy is a procedure in which a surgical incision is made in the tissues of the birth canal just before the baby's head is born. This cut causes trauma to the woman's genital region, requires stitches after the birth, and is a matter that is considered a violation of the woman's human rights amongst natural childbirth advocates.

The World Health Organization (WHO) states,

"Limiting the use of episiotomy to strict indications has a number of benefits: less...trauma, less need for suturing and fewer complications.... Routine episiotomy, or liberal use of episiotomy, is unfortunately very common, both in under-resourced settings and in some developed countries....There are...strong reasons to counteract the overuse of episiotomy..."

Many Obstetrics Behind the Times

This medical intervention has been done routinely for decades. However, those who stay current with scientific research have all but abandoned the procedure. Sadly, I find it lingering on as a matter of routine in the practice of several of the local obstetricians I have personally spoken to. I also receive similar feedback from many of my clients who have asked me about the procedure after discussing it with their doctors in both Saudi Arabia and in Egypt.

East vs. West

Although too many women are still being cut in the West, there is growing consumerism in this regard, as women have become educated on the subject over the past years. These women seek out doctors who do not cut as a matter of routine and often refuse the procedure all together. However, in Arabia I find that most doctors still cut routinely and the local women simply accept the cut as a matter of fact, barely giving the issue a second thought.

I recently discovered a blatant illustration of the differing practice of the West and Middle East in this regards. First, while watching a Canadian midwifery training video, the instructor was displaying the many instruments that may be used during birth. When she came to episiotomy scissors she made a side comment, *"I know nobody does episiotomies anymore, but we have to carry them in case of an emergency."*

I was almost in tears as I heard her make that statement so casually. Her words rang through my head as I recalled my interactions with obstetricians in Egypt and Saudi Arabia. I practically cried as I thought to myself, *"If only that were the case over here!"*

My memory of conversations on this side of the globe include:

"Aisha, truly, you are special to have never had an episiotomy..." counseled my obstetrician in Egypt after discussing the matter during one of my pre-natal visits.

"One hundred percent of first-time mothers must have an episiotomy," confidently declared a doctor in a Saudi clinic.

"My doctor told me Arab women have less collagen in their skin than Western women and therefore always need to be cut," lamented one of my childbirth students in Riyadh. (I would have liked to ask the doctor for the scientific proof to back that up!)

This is not to say that ALL doctors in the West are good nor all in the East are bad. You can find both categories everywhere. But I think it's accurate to say that more doctors routinely cut in Arabia than in the West.

But I haven't lost faith. I was pleased to find an article by **Joanna Hartley** in the UAE, "Hospital Slashes Episiotomy Rate," which provides a ray of hope in the Middle East. I also know of at least one local hospital midwife who doesn't cut as a mater of routine, *masha'Allah*.

Ignoring the Evidence

I don't even want to think of how many women around the globe are cut during their births as a matter of course. From my perspective, this is a tragedy, as there is plenty of scientific evidence that indicates that the intervention should be used sparingly, not routinely.

I recently asked a local hospital midwife about her experience with Arab women, as my student's doctor commenting about there being a difference in skin texture had me perplexed. She told me that in her fifteen years as a delivering midwife in Saudi, she has not seen any difference between the anatomies of Arab women as compared to Westerners. She said the need for episiotomy should come down to individual assessment of the elasticity of the tissues, the size of the baby, how much physical preparation the _Mother_ has done in this regards for her birth, the control with which she is pushing, and the caregivers skill at assisting the woman to birth without significant tearing of the tissues. In her personal practice, she has found no difference based on ethnicity or race alone.

In fact, I feel that any doctor who says that 100% (or any other high number) of women of any category (first-time _Mothers_, Arabs, etc.) need an episiotomy is simply treating patients as a matter of protocol. It's quite obvious that such a doctor is not treating each woman as an individual, nor assessing the situation on an individual basis. Personally, I'd run in the opposite direction from such a doctor, as I feel that birth should be cared for on an individual basis and not as a matter of routine.

My Perspective Cut vs. Tear

When I teach childbirth classes, I give women specific postures and exercises to increase the elasticity of the subject tissues and I discuss with them the risk of tearing if an episiotomy is refused.

The way I see it is that an episiotomy is a guaranteed trauma with a need for stitches and painful healing after birth; whereas taking the risk of tearing gives a possibility of no trauma at all, or slightly mild trauma, which may not even need stitching (minor skin laceration).

Even if the woman tears significantly, it's usually not any worse than had she been cut. Of course, doctors may argue that a straight cut is easier to repair, but frankly, I am more concerned with the woman's wellbeing than I am ensuring that the doctor has an easy job!

Another common retort by obstetricians is that a cut will control the direction of the tear. Again, without a cut, she may not tear at all and with a cut there is a weakening of the tissue integrity that often leads to a tear that extends the incision even further.

Additionally, I have a personal friend who confided that she had an episiotomy with her first birth and she refused one for her second. With the second birth she encountered the dreaded upwards tear. She told me that the pain from the tear, even though it was in a much more sensitive area, was far less than the previous episiotomy. She had no regrets about refusing the procedure for her second birth.

Ways to Prepare

So this leaves me to counsel you on what you can do to avoid being cut during birth. The American Academy of Husband-Coached Childbirth® publishes a paper titled *"What can I do to avoid an episiotomy?"* It includes several tips for expectant mothers. I've listed them here, along with a few of my own:

1. *Good Nutrition* to ensure healthy tissue elasticity.

2. *Squatting Exercises* to stretch the tissues before birth.

3. *Exposure to Air* to keep the tissues healthy.

4. *Daily Kegel Exercises* (see Chapter 14).

5. *Avoid Soap* as it dries tissues (cleanse with plain water instead).

6. *Lotion and Massage* to soften tissues and help mother become comfortable with her own anatomy.

7. *Talk to Your Doctor in Advance* about your desires and preparations to avoid episiotomy.

8. *Be Patient* during birth. An episiotomy can speed up the delivery by a few contractions, but it isn't worth the resulting pain and recovery trauma.

9. *Pull Your Knees Back (or Squat)* during birth. Do not spread your legs wide open (which also means stay out of stirrups!).

10. *Push With Self Control* at the moment of birth to ensure you gently ease the baby's head out and stop for the shoulders to naturally rotate during the subsequent contraction.

11. *Remind Your Doctor at the Time of Birth*; don't assume they recall

your wishes in this regards (also have your companion watch and advocate for no cuts during the birth).

12. ***Don't Take Medicinal Pain Relief***, as it prevents you from being able to push with self control.

Notes of Exception

It is important to note that in cases of emergency (such as a baby in severe distress or in need of assisted delivery with vacuum extraction or forceps) an episiotomy may be warranted. But such instances are rare.

Also, for women who have undergone female circumcision, their case should be evaluated carefully to determine if the procedure significantly altered the opening of the birth canal or the available elasticity of the tissues.

Additionally, for those women that opt for epidural or other medicinal pain relief, they should consider the fact that their inability to feel the pushing phase of their birth may result in increased incidence of severe tearing as they are not able to assess how strongly to push, nor can they sense the moment the head passes through the opening to stop their pushing and await rotation of the shoulders. They are therefore more likely to inadvertently injure themselves with uncontrolled pushing.

Conclusion

In the end, your doctor has the most power over whether or not you will be cut. Your job includes:

1. Educating yourself on how to prepare your body so that you don't "need" the cut.

2. Be a good consumer by finding a doctor who does not routinely cut.

3. Learning how to cope with your labor and birth without medicinal pain relief so that you can push with self-control when the time comes.

In the end, you are the one who has to live with the consequences of your birth experience. Whether or not you have an episiotomy is not the end of the world, but it will surely make a difference in how you feel about your birth as well as how much pain and healing you'll need to do afterwards.

Hemorrhoids

Some *Mothers* suffer hemorrhoids from pushing too hard during birth. These are burst blood vessels in or around the anus. They may appear like small clusters of grapes. They are very painful and sometimes itch. Kegel exercises (see Chapter 14) help to avoid them and heal them faster if they do appear. Sitting in a shallow water (sitz) bath to soak the area keeps it clean and provides some relief.

Applying pharmaceutical hemorrhoid creams or suppositories usually provide great relief. The active ingredient in many pharmaceutical remedies is Hamamelis Virginiana, better known as Witch Hazel. Many women prefer to make their own distilled liquid, ointment, or medicated pads from the herb. Hemorrhoids typically heal within a week or so, however, in rare but severe cases, surgery is recommended.

Postpartum Rest

The biggest issue with many natural birth *Mothers* is the tendency to forget that they actually need a recovery period. These women feel so good after birth that they may overdo things and fail to slow down as much as needed. Aside from craving a really good meal and needing some well-deserved rest after birth, they feel terrific.

It is important, however, that every new *Mother* and baby have some quiet downtime to get to know each other and establish a good breastfeeding relationship. This takes practice, patience, determination, and time.

In fact, in many cultures it is customary for the new *Mother* to be pampered and excused of any activity outside of caring for her new baby for up to forty days. I think this is a terrific practice, so long as it doesn't include someone else bottle feeding her baby so she can rest. It's important that she spend this time with the baby to establish exclusive breastfeeding.

Honestly, most women who birth all naturally don't physically need to be taken care of, although extra time and attention is surely nice and there's certainly nothing wrong with the practice. But I sincerely pray that you feel so good after birth that you don't require such pampering, though you may choose to indulge in it anyway.

Cesarean Recovery

Approximately ten percent of women will truly need a surgical delivery to ensure the health and safety of theirs and/or their baby's lives. For those _Mothers_ I have included an article from my Saudi Life Motherhood column, "After Cesarean Tips:"

After Cesarean Tips

KEEP in mind that I don't recommend surgical birth, except in the event of true life or death complications. However, I want to provide tips for better healing for the population of _Mothers_ who will find themselves faced with Cesarean deliveries.

Since I have not experienced Cesarean first-hand (_alhamdulillah_), I've done some research and asked around to compile this list of tips. Please feel free to add your suggestions in the comment section.

Even _Mothers_ who are not intending on Cesarean can benefit from these tips "just in case" they find themselves faced with this type of birth. I truly feel, "knowledge is power," and the more prepared you are for all possibilities, the better your birth experience will be.

Emotional Advice

Many _Mothers_ feel disheartened when a natural birth plan turns surgical. It is well known that postpartum depression is much more prevalent after Cesarean delivery. Don't feel ashamed if you feel you may be suffering from PPD. Birth and the postpartum period are times of hormonal and emotional ups and downs (even when everything does go according to plan). It's important that you find someone to talk to about your feelings. (If you are the loved one of a woman you suspect may be suffering from PPD, don't ignore the issue. It's important that she get help to regain her emotional stability and ability to care for herself and her new baby.) Always remember:

1. Trust *Allah's* decree for your birth.

2. Make the most of the experience, regardless of the method.

3. Your baby's birth will forever be a special memory.

4. Keep your focus on the baby and make mental note of his/her beautiful appearance.

5. Once a decision is made, take confidence that you are doing what you feel is best for the health and safety of both mom and baby.

6. Talk about your feelings with someone you trust.

Physical Advice

Perhaps the most frustrating part of surgical delivery is the recovery period afterwards. Cesarean can leave *Mothers* weak, nauseous, and in pain for weeks. The drugs used to control pain can make breastfeeding more challenging as baby may be too groggy to nurse and *Mother's* milk supply can be affected by the medications. Below are some tips from moms who have been there:

1. Walk as soon as you can after surgery (start slowly).

2. Hold a pillow over your incision when coughing, sneezing, laughing, or holding your baby.

3. Sometimes there is congestion in the lungs from the anesthesia. Splash rubbing alcohol on the back and then firmly tap/slap the upper back to loosen the phlegm and make it easier to cough.

4. Eat lightly to avoid gas pains.

5. Drink plenty of liquids.

6. Drink beverages at room temperature (avoid hot or cold drinks).

7. Do not use drinking straws (the sucking action tugs at your incision).

8. A belly wrap may help to support the incision site while healing.

9. Get help around the house, do not bend to pick up anything and do not lift anything other than the baby.

10. Eat a balanced diet with lots of fresh fruits, vegetables, and whole grain foods to keep your bowels smooth; avoid foods that constipate (cheese, fried foods, sweets, starches, etc.)

11. Lay flat on your back, and occasionally on your stomach with a pillow under your incision.

12. Surgical delivery eliminates the baby's exposure to important live cultures in the birth canal (probiotics), therefore it is extremely important that Cesarean born infants are breastfed exclusively. (For more information read Infant Health Benefits from Natural Birth and Breastfeeding in Chapter 29.)

13. If you have a childbirth teacher or doula, discuss your concerns or problems with her (yes, call her even it's the middle of the night!).

Above all, cherish the newborn time, it passes quickly and before you know it your baby's infancy and your pain will be a fading memory. May Allah bless all mothers and babies with safe, gentle birth experiences!

Postpartum Bleeding

Most women will bleed for about forty days after the birth of their baby. The bleeding should noticeably decrease by the third to fifth day and the color will begin to change from bright red to pink and finally to a yellowish or white color. If you are soaking more than one large feminine pad per hour or your blood remains very bright red beyond the first week you are bleeding abnormally or too much and should consult your doctor. If blood becomes a bright red after it had changed to a lighter color, it is a sign you are being too active and you need to take it easy.

Excused of *Islamic* Duties Due to Postpartum Bleeding

Blood from the womb is considered postnatal blood if it is related to the birth of a child, whether alive or stillborn. If the pregnancy ends in miscarriage before there are visual signs of human features, it is not considered postpartum bleeding, this is usually the case when the pregnancy ends during the first eighty to ninety days of the pregnancy.

Islamic scholars agree that during the time of postpartum bleeding, a woman is excused from obligatory prayers and the fasting of *Ramadan*. Actually, they are more than excused, for even if they were to make *salat* or fast, it would not count. The prayers she misses during this time do not need to be made up later, however, any days of missed fasting during the month of *Ramadan* do need to be made up.

In addition, she may not have sexual intercourse at this time. This does not mean that she cannot be close to or intimate with her husband, so long as their intimacy avoids sexual penetration. Also, she may not make *tawaf* (ritual circumambulation of the *Ka'bah in Makkah*), touch the *Qur'an*, be declared divorced, or stay in the *masjid*.

It's important to note that touching the *Qur'an* during menstruation and postpartum bleeding is a point of disagreement amongst *Muslim* scholars. The popular opinion in Saudi Arabia is that it is forbidden, however there are scholars who state that it's permissible to touch the *Qur'an* based on the fact that no explicit proof exists from the *Qur'an* or *Sunnah* regarding its prohibition, though it's certainly *mustahabb* (highly recommended) to be in *wudhu* when touching the *Qur'an*. Others say that it's okay to handle the *Qur'an* with a barrier, such as gloves, during this time.

Some *Muslims* believe a woman cannot even read, without touching, or recite verses of *Qur'an* from memory during this time. However, according to Shaikh Ibn Baz, *Grand Mufti* of Saudi Arabia, this is incorrect, as he says that it is important they continue to read, without touching the *Qur'an*, and recite so that they do not lose what they have memorized and it is also permissible to read books of supplication that have verses of *Qur'an* and *hadith* mixed in.

As for the term of her postpartum excuse, there are differing opinions amongst the scholars. However, most agree that it begins as soon as she sees blood related to the childbirth, whether before, during, or after the actual birth and ends with the cessation of such bleeding. Most scholars agree that there is no minimum time and in rare cases, where the _Mother_ experiences no birth related bleeding, she must continue her obligatory duties without ceasing. However, there is slight disagreement regarding the maximum term of postpartum excuse. The _Hanafi_, _Maliki_, and _Hanbali_ schools of thought concur that the maximum period of postpartum excuse is forty days, and in most cases the _Mother_ will stop bleeding by this time. There are some conflicting ideas that the maximum term is sixty days.

When your postpartum bleeding ceases, or you have reached the maximum time of excuse, you must perform _ghusl_ (complete ablution by bathing and ritual cleansing) before resuming your _Islamic_ obligations. If you are resuming prayers due to reaching the maximum term but are still bleeding, you must make _ghusl_ and wear a protective feminine pad while praying and you must make _wudhu_ before every prayer while in this state.

The issue of _Islamic fiqh_ (law) with regard to obligatory duties is extremely important. I am sharing this information with you from what I believe to be reliable sources, but I must disclose that I am not an _Islamic_ scholar. Fortunately, we are blessed to have knowledgeable scholars alive and around us and we can always consult them if we have questions or concerns regarding these issues or any conflicting opinions. Anything good in this advice is from _Allah_ and any error is my own.

Chapter 12

The Baby's Needs and Rights

Sometimes the forgotten partner in birth is the baby. The intensity of the _Mother's_ sensations leaves her totally withdrawn and focused inward. After the birth she may be understandably exhausted or may have been so traumatized that she just wants to escape the whole scene and get the last steps over with.

Where does this leave the baby? Many delivery room attendants have said that the _Mothers_ don't want their babies right away. They push them away and want a moment to themselves, before dealing with the baby, or they don't want the baby until it's been cleaned up and dressed. So who do you think is going to cuddle, love, and reassure YOUR baby in those initial moments in the cold bright world?

Hopefully, the nurses who tend to your baby may have a degree of compassion and gentleness for your baby. But honestly, they do this day in and day out. No one LOVES your baby like you do. Also, they are required to keep physical barriers between themselves and the babies to avoid the possibility of spreading disease from bodily fluids.

If ever I could scream, "Wake up _Mothers_!" it would be in those precious moments after birth. Bring your baby into your arms and up to your chest right away. Warm him/her against your bare chest and allow him/her to hear the familiar beat of your heart that has been the rhythm of the world for the past nine months. So what if the baby is "dirty" or even bloody. You can wash later! You will never get a second chance to soothe your baby into the world. These first moments will make a lasting impression on how your child sees the world. Is it a gentle loving place where he/she can trust to have all his/her needs met? Or is it a cold bright place full of rough surfaces, rubber gloves, strange voices, and distant handling? What do you want for your newborn baby?

There are gentler options, there are more natural options, there are better options to what is routine in most hospital settings.

Gentler Options

AMANI Birth looks for gentle alternatives to the way women, babies, and families are treated during pregnancy, labor and birth. Most families just aren't aware that gentler alternatives exist. Educating families about their options and helping them prepare and stay healthy and low risk is just the first step.

Unfortunately, we are a long way away from the family centered birthing of our ancestors where woman-to-woman care and sharing birth experiences was the norm. In fact, in today's medicalized birthing culture, few women have ever seen a birth before having their own. As a culture, women are left with few options besides handing their bodies over to the medical institution like a car to a mechanic. They don't know what to expect, what choices they have, or how those choices will ultimately affect them, their babies, their families, and ultimately the world in which we live.

Birthing Routines

The heartbreak with normal routines carried out at most births is that so many are unnecessary. They are performed as a matter of protocol without assessing need. Sadly, many of these procedures are traumatizing as well as physically and emotionally harmful. In fact, leading organizations like ACOG and WHO have even removed many of these routines from their recommended list of protocols (episiotomy, infant suctioning, immediate cord clamping, etc.), yet they are still done day after day to the detriment of our women and babies.

One example is the routine cutting of women during delivery (episiotomy, see Chapter 11). There are so many advantages to allowing the baby to be born on an intact perineum (this means NOT cutting the mother down below). The squeezing of the baby that therefore takes place rids him/her of fluid in the lungs naturally, and suctioning becomes virtually unnecessary. Also, _Mother_ is typically able to birth without the cut, and even if she tears, most will be minor skin tissue tears, as compared to muscles that are cut by well-meaning birth attendants.

Suctioning a baby as a matter of routine, rather than need, is barbaric. Babies should be born and directly placed on _Mother's_ bare chest, skin-to-skin, for immediate bonding and breastfeeding. All of the routine protocols performed on babies at birth can either wait, be performed on _Mother's_ chest, or be abandoned all together.

The _Mother's_ oxytocin levels (hormones that stimulate loving feelings) will never be stronger than the period immediately following birth. _Allah_ (_SWT_) has provided us with this flood of hormones to solidify our bonding care for our infants.

Additionally, our infants have just come from a warm, dark, quiet environment. The way he/she transitions into the world will have lifelong effects on his/her fragile personality. What better way to facilitate this change than to be placed in the warm, loving arms of _Mother_ whose warm milk smells of the watery environment from which he came and soothing sweet taste of her breast milk (colostrum) provides the first boost of antibodies and immunities the baby needs to thrive and survive?

This golden first hour after birth is especially precious and _Mothers_ and babies should never be separated or interrupted during that time unless the baby is in a dire state, and even then, his/her best chance for recovery is on mother's chest. Kangaroo care (babies held skin-to-skin on _Mother's_ chest) has proven to be more valuable for babies in distress than any baby-warming incubator. In fact, a very well documented and researched clinical guideline, with 167 references, urges implementation of kangaroo care and appeared in the June 2008 issue of Advances in Neonatal Care. It simply goes against the scientific evidence to whisk the baby away from mother immediately after birth, and yet, tragically, this is what routinely happens in many hospitals throughout the world.

Islamic Rights

Another tragic side effect of hospital routines that separate _Mother_ and baby is the lost opportunity for the baby's first auditory experience to be of one of his/her parents calling the *athan* in his or her right ear and the *iqamah* in his or her left ear.

In *Sahih Bukhari* [4:506] it is narrated, **"When any human being is born, Satan pinches the body with his two fingers, except 'Isa, the son of Maryam, whom Satan tried to pinch but failed, for he touched the placenta instead."**

Knowing this, don't you want to protect your child and do as the Prophet (*Sallallaahu 'alayhi wa sallam*) did? Abu Raf'I relates, **"I saw the Prophet [Sallallaahu 'alayhi wa sallam] saying the athan of salah in the ear of his grandson, Hasan, when the child was born to his daughter, Fatima."** This *hadith* is found in *Musnad Ahmad*, and authenticated by Shaikh Abdul Qadir 'Arnaut.

Reciting the *athan* in the right ear is considered a stronger *hadith* than that of calling the *iqamah* in the left. However, I was able to find more information about this and feel comfortable in recommending it. This is a direct quote from an article titled "_Proof of Giving Athan and iqamah in Newborn Baby's Ear_":

> *Hafiz Ibn al-Qayyim, in his valuable book on the regulations relating to the newborn Tuhfat al-Mawdud bi-Ahkam al-Mawlud, has included a chapter entitled "Concerning the desirability of giving athan in the newborn's right ear, and iqamah in the left." He cites three hadiths on the subject (of varying authenticities), and then proceeds to point out some of the possible deeper meaning and rationale behind this practice: that it is wise to ensure that the first words the baby hears are*

words containing the majesty and greatness of Allah, and a reminder of the testimony of faith by which one enters Islam, and with which one would be reminded by other Muslims close to one's death. We also know (as narrated by Muslim) that every human being has one of the jinn accompanying him, and calling athan to the newborn ensures that the call to goodness and true faith precedes the whisperings to evil that would later come from the accompanying devil. It is also established (as narrated by Bukhari and Muslim) that Satan runs away from athan, and this reveals a further benefit.

Although this can be performed later, of course, it is so much more reassuring to know that you are immediately protecting the faith of your newborn child through this practice. Abu Hurairah reported: "**The Messenger of Allah (Sallallaahu 'alayhi wa sallam), said, "No one is born except they are upon natural instinct [Islam]; then his parents turn him into a Jew or Christian or Magian."**

AMANI Birth Centers

AMANI Birth seeks to help women put an end to such damaging procedures, one birth at a time. It's our vision to have specialized AMANI Birth Centers where each individual case is treated based on true need and these types of harmful and non evidence based protocols simply won't exist, *in sha' Allah*.

Parent education must be our top priority so that expectant couples can advocate for themselves in our current birthing culture. Next must be widespread awareness for birth attendants, including AMANI Birth friendly attendants and birthplace certifications, *in sha'Allah*. In our first phase, including publication of this book and live AMANI Birth classes, it's parent education that must precede everything else. Through the awakening of our *Mothers* will come the demand for changes in practice that will afford better, gentle births for our babies, *in sha'Allah*.

CHAPTER 13

What to Expect in <u>AMANI Birth</u> Training-Part Two

The <u>Mothers</u> Series focuses on the "Power of Knowledge." Although we encourage <u>Mothers</u> to choose her birth companions and advocate for team training, it's important for her to know that she will birth with or without her partner(s). She should therefore have the confidence to do it alone, just in case she finds herself in a situation to do so. Lone birthing is not our ideal, however, <u>Mothers</u> are beautifully strong and can make it through!

 Understanding how your body works in labor and birth will help you best prepare for the big day. Knowing your options and weighing them thoroughly ahead of time will allow you to prioritize and make the decisions that you feel best for your new family. Knowing what to expect will help you remain calm as you anticipate each stage of your labor. With preparation and a calm attitude towards birth it truly can be the most joyful and empowering event of a woman's life, *in sha' Allah*. Perhaps the most important piece is preparing mentally and emotionally for <u>Mothering</u> the new baby.

The <u>Mothers</u> series is compiled of four modules:

Module 1   Physiology of Pregnancy

In this module we will explore the physiology of pregnancy and the changes that occur in the _Mother's_ body during this special time of her life. We will observe the many built in safeguards for the unborn baby and examine the stages of gestation. The importance of assuming responsibility as "primary care provider" for the baby will be discussed. We also provide a guide to many of the common discomforts in pregnancy, their causes, and relief measures to try.

Module 2   Stages of Labor

This module will ensure familiarity with the three phases of labor including an in depth look at the special challenges of transitioning between the first and second stages. We will explore how the body works during labor to ensure the _Mother_ is best prepared to work with her body to minimize pain and discomfort, _in sha'Allah_. We will review Braxton Hicks (practice) contractions as well as what "real" labor feels like. We will discuss how to time contractions and explore normal variations during natural labors.

Module 3   Overview of Labor and Birth

This module will include an in depth focus on what to expect in labor and various options _Mothers_ can choose based on their personal research and preferences. _Mother_-led pushing, delayed cord clamping, and kangaroo care are discussed as important considerations in natural births.

Module 4   Postpartum Care

This module will discuss the normal postnatal period for new _Mothers_. We will review warning signs of problems and when to call your caregiver as well as the importance of good nutrition and rest in healing after birth. The role of breastfeeding in the maternal healing process will also be explored as well as postnatal exercise and other topics for after birth, including the _Islamic fiqh_ (law) of postpartum bleeding.

Part Three - _Active_

When we look to the _Qur'an_ for any reference to labor and birth we find the story of Maryam's/Mary's (_Alayhas-Salam_) birth of Isa/Jesus (_Alayhis-Salām_). Some things to note from her account:

- She found a quiet place of seclusion, away from the peering observational eyes of strangers.

- Allah sent to her a stream to cool her eye and quench her thirst.

- She shook the date tree, which indicates her upright, _Active_ position with freedom of movement.

- She ate dates for energy as she labored.

And [when] the throes of childbirth drove her to the trunk of a palm-tree, she exclaimed: "Oh, would that I had died ere this, and had become a thing forgotten, utterly forgotten!" Thereupon [a voice] called out to her from beneath that [palm-tree]: "Grieve not! Thy Sustainer has provided a rivulet [running] beneath thee; and shake the trunk of the palm-tree towards thee: it will drop fresh, ripe dates upon thee. Eat, then, and drink, and let thine eye be gladdened! And if thou shouldst see any human being, convey this unto him: `Behold, abstinence from speech have I vowed unto the Most Gracious; hence, I may not speak today to any mortal. [Qur'an 19:23-26]

Allah (SWT), in His infinite wisdom, provided us this scene as our only direct reference to labor and birth. How different is this than the current day tether to an IV line with doctor's orders of "nothing by mouth?" All the while we strap mothers to fetal monitors that keep women immobile and lying in bed to labor, often times flat on their backs.

<u>AMANI Birth</u> follows many of its predecessors in challenging the hospital mantra of "nothing by mouth and lying flat on your back in stirrups for delivery." Ancient artifacts, recent scientific evidence, and *Islamic* history all paint a very different picture of birth.

In this section we will discuss the importance of exercise and good nutrition to prepare for the birthing event as well as following our natural instincts to stay *Active* and nourished during labor and birth. Of course, it's no surprise that our model of birth may be different from many hospitals', as we advocate the power of women to birth their babies, whereas hospitals advocate the power of doctors to deliver them – and *Allah* knows best.

CHAPTER 14

Pregnancy Nutrition and Exercise

As I learned from Dr. Bradley's work, birth is an athletic event. In fact it may well be one of the most challenging events in a woman's life. *Allah (SWT)* has given us the gift of ample time before birth to prepare, *alhamdulillah*. It would be foolish of us to waste this time and expect that the heroes in white (or blue) coats will rush in at the last minute to "save" us from our own lax ignorance.

Physically speaking, a woman will exert the type of energy used in running a marathon or, as Dr. Bradley used to say, swimming a mile (1.6 kilometers) during her labor and birth. If you were told that in a few months time you would be thrown into deep water, wouldn't it be reckless not to prepare?

The energy and muscles exertion needed to birth takes strength, determination, focus, and stamina. Most of us are not living lives that are conducive to this type of physical activity. But the good news is: we have several months notice before the event to prepare and plan for success. Make good use of this time to improve your diet, exercise your muscles, and improve flexibility so that you can come to the start line ready to give it all you've got in order to cross the finish line in best form, *in sha' Allah*.

Nutrition

Speaking first of nutrition, eating well is the single most important thing you can do for your baby right now. In fact, only you can control what goes into your body and your baby on a daily basis. Keep in mind your body is providing all the nutrients and materials to build a new human being from single drops of fluid. Your baby is literally being built from virtually nothing from the foods you eat.

"He creates man out of a [mere] drop of sperm..." [Qur'an 6:4]

Allah (SWT) has given the expectant mother a huge charge of trust and responsibility in bringing forth new life. We can best honor this trust by avoiding junk food and eating a balanced diet every single day. Keeping our intentions on honoring *Allah* is one way we can worship HIM through the simple act of eating, *in sha'Allah.*

During my training as a doula, childbirth educator, and midwife the recommendations of Dr. Thomas Brewer have come up time and again as the foremost expert on pregnancy nutrition. In <u>Metabolic Toxemia of Late Pregnancy</u> he shares his research for helping women stay healthy during pregnancy and keeping low-risk through nutrition.

Obviously, a balanced diet is needed for all of us to maintain good health and balance in our bodies. However, it is especially important during pregnancy when our babies are depending on us to provide everything needed for the formation of complete body systems.

I can't stress enough how important it is to consistently eat well, as your baby is not a parasite and does not take from your stores of nutrients as was once thought. The baby gets all it's energy sources directly from the mother's circulating blood. This means that only that which she has inhaled, ingested or injected reaches the placenta for transmission to the baby.

Dr. Brewer wrote of not only the importance of balance in your diet, but also avoiding empty calories and junk food. What's more, his research showed that lack of protein was the biggest health threat for expectant women. According to his findings and subsequent studies thereafter, pregnant women should consume over 75 grams of protein daily to protect against metabolic toxemia, one of the most dreaded pregnancy induced illnesses.

His diet recommendations are covered in more depth in the <u>AMANI Birth</u> classes, but can also easily be found by Internet search online.

One other important point to note, weight gain during pregnancy is much less indicative of good health as is monitoring the foods which are eaten to gain that weight. There is a range of "normal" when it comes to weight gain and each woman comes into pregnancy in various degrees of "shape" to start with. Putting too much focus on "how much" is gained is far less productive than learning "how to eat well."

For some specifics about the importance of vitamins in terms of a healthy increase in blood volume during pregnancy and efficient clotting of blood after birth, I have included an article from my Saudi Life Motherhood column, Blood, Pregnancy, and Nutrition":

Blood, Pregnancy, and Nutrition

EVERYONE is aware that absence of a woman's menses is one of the first signs of pregnancy. But the more I study about the physiology of pregnancy and birth, the more I've come to appreciate the role of our blood during this miraculous time in our lives. I've also come to realize the importance of our nutrition in maintaining the health and function of our blood.

Increased Volume

First of all, the volume of the blood in the woman's body is increased by about 50% during pregnancy. This is reflective of *Allah's* perfect design, as we will shed blood after the birth our babies. If it weren't for this natural increase in blood volume, the blood loss could otherwise compromise our life.

Yet, this natural safety net may not be fully present for all women. It is inherent by design; however, nutrition makes a huge contribution to maximizing this increase in volume.

Most everyone is aware of the importance of iron to our blood. But did you know that iron is not absorbed very well by the body in the presence of calcium? This means, if you take an iron pill with milk, or eat iron rich foods with cheese, for example, you are not getting the full benefit of the iron.

Conversely, iron is absorbed best in the presence of vitamin C. So consider taking your iron supplements with orange juice and eating your iron rich foods in conjunction with vitamin C foods. It's also important to realize that the body does not store vitamin C, making daily consumption essential.

There are other considerations that are important for maintaining a healthy blood volume as well. Some of these include an adequate intake of water and salt. **Therefore, it's important to follow your body's cues and drink to thirst and salt your food to taste.**

Blood Doesn't Mix

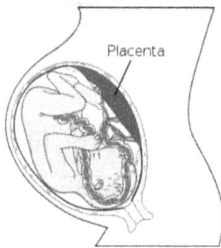

Placenta

Source: Wikipedia

Another intriguing point is that the mother's blood and the baby's blood don't mix in the womb. The placenta is a magnificent organ that manages nutrient and waste exchange between the mother and her baby. It is also the only organ that is grown as needed and disposed of after use, *subhan'Allah*.

The function of the placenta is to receive blood from the mother's circulation on its maternal side, and excrete oxygen and dietary nutrients. It then passes them to the baby's side, where the baby's blood is infused through the umbilical cord with these vital components of life.

At the same time, the placenta excretes the baby's waste on the baby's side and passes them to the mother's side, where the mother's blood carries the waste through her circulatory system to be eliminated.

The mother must take extreme care in what she ingests, inhales, or injects into her body. Most everything that enters her blood stream crosses the placenta and reaches the baby within 60 seconds. This places great responsibility on the mother to be cautious with her diet and environment.

Blood Clotting

As mentioned above, a woman will undoubtedly lose blood after the birth of her baby. Along with the increased blood volume is the safety feature of our blood to clot in an effort to control bleeding. If the blood does not clot efficiently, the woman can easily suffer a postpartum hemorrhage, which is a leading cause of maternal death.

What most people don't realize is the role of nutrition in the blood's ability to clot. Our blood simply cannot clot in the absence of calcium and vitamin K. If our stores of calcium are low, our body will dig into any reserves in our bones, thereby weakening them. With this in mind, it is imperative that women consume adequate amounts of calcium and vitamin K during their pregnancy to ensure the blood's maximum ability to clot. Not to mention the very important role that calcium plays on the development of teeth and bones in the developing baby.

Dietary Sources

The essential vitamins and minerals, noted above, are not produced by the body. They must be consumed. Below is a small list of some their sources. It is recommended that you do your own research and determine foods that will help you maximize your health.

Vitamin K	Calcium (Absorbed w/Vit D)	Vitamin C (Not Stored)	Iron (Eat w/ Vitamin C)
Spinach	Milk/Cheese/Dairy	Citrus Fruits	Beans
Green Beans	Almonds	Strawberries	Seeds/Nuts
Carrots	Okra	Bell Peppers	Red Meat
Grapes	Sesame Seeds	Parsley	Leafy Vegetables
Broccoli	Broccoli	Broccoli	Dried Fruits
Asparagus	Egg Whites	Tomatoes	Eggs Yolks
Pharmacy Supplements	Pharmacy Supplements	Pharmacy Supplements	Pharmacy Supplements

Nutrition plays a major role in the health of the woman and baby. It is also a huge component in the safety of the birth. What's more, it is the single greatest factor that a pregnant woman has control over.

Trust *Allah* and tie your camels by learning what you can do to ensure the inherent safety of birth is maximized for you and your baby. May *Allah* grant you good health during your pregnancy and beyond!

No Redos

One thing to realize is that there are no "redos" in human development. *Allah* has prepared the blueprint for our development in the womb that dictates when each part of the body is formed and determines precisely when specific growth patterns occur:

> *"...We create man out of the essence of clay, and then We cause him to remain as a drop of sperm in [the wombs] firm keeping, and then We create out of the drop of sperm a germ-cell, and then We create out of the germ-cell an embryonic lump, and then We create within the embryonic lump bones, and then We clothe the bones with flesh - and then We bring [all] this into being as a new creation hallowed, therefore, is God, the best of artisans!"* [Qur'an 23:12-14]

We know that the first three months are the greatest in terms of rapid division of cells, as well as development of tissues, organs, and body systems. From this point on the growth rate is still phenomenal when compared to the rate of growth and development outside the womb.

Because every moment of every day during pregnancy is an explosion of growth, it is imperative that the mother consistently consumes the nutrients needed to support and maximize the baby's growth and development potential. This is not to say that a slack in diet will necessarily make a noticeable difference, but then again, there is no way to go back and compare the baby's development against what it would have or could have been had the mother eaten better at the precise moment of any specific developing tissue.

The baby cannot make up for deficits in growth that occur in the womb. Growth after birth is not the same as growth in utero. In order to maximize the baby's inherent potential, we must provide a steady stream of nutrients and also allow the uncomplicated pregnancy to go to full term.

Variety is Key

Allah (SWT) provided us a wide variety of foods to choose from. Picking from among the good foods and maintaining a variety in your diet is the best way to ensure that you are getting everything needed to grow a healthy baby, *in sha' Allah.*

> *"He created cattle that give you warmth, benefits, and food to eat."* (Qur'an 16:5)

> *"...and from it (the earth) we produced grain for their sustenance."* (Qur'an 36:33)

> *"It is He who sends down water from the sky with which He brings up corn, olives, dates and grapes and other fruit."* (Qur'an 16:11)

> *"And it is He Who produces gardens and crops of different shape and taste (its fruits and its seeds) and olives, and pomegranates, similar (in kind) and different (in taste). Eat of their fruit when they ripen..."* (Qur'an 6:141)

> *"In cattle too you have a worthy lesson. We give you to drink of that which is in their bellies...pure milk, a pleasant beverage for those who drink it."* (Qur'an 16:66)

> *"It is He who subdued the seas, from which you eat fresh fish."* (Qur'an 16:14)

Key Points

- *Allah* Provides What We Need

  - ➤ Foods are the natural form of nutrition and best assimilated by the body.

  - ➤ Everyday foods supply essential nutrients for pregnancy and baby.

  - ➤ *Allah* has built in many safety nets for pregnancy and birth.

- Complete Nutrition is Important

  - ➤ Herbs are foods that can be an added source of vitamins and minerals.

  - ➤ Ample caloric intake (+/-3000) is necessary for proper body function.

  - ➤ Pregnancy is a time to focus on eating right, not for focus on the scale.

- Variety is Key to a Healthy Pregnancy and Best Start for Baby

  - ➤ A good assortment of elements ensures the best outcomes.

  - ➤ Various nutrients, vitamins, and minerals work best together.

  - ➤ Utilizing the many *halal* foods *Allah* provided is a form of worship.

- Special Circumstances Require Special Consideration

  - ➤ Smoking and illnesses may decrease the body's ability to process foods.

  - ➤ Pharmaceutical supplements may be used in rare cases of deficiency.

  - ➤ Vegetarian/vegans/lactose intolerant, etc. need to pay particular attention to elements typically derived from meat and dairy sources.

- *"Tie your camel" -* Good Nutrition Maximizes Built in Safeties

  - ➤ Replace processed/fast/"junk" foods with fresher/healthier choices

  - ➤ Honey and fruits can be good substitutes for sweets.

Exercise

Birth will take strength, stamina, and flexibility. Every pregnant woman should be getting some form of regular exercise daily. Walking and swimming are simple and good regimens for strength and stamina. Walking is especially easy, as it doesn't require any special knowledge, skills, or equipment. In fact, walking opens the inlet of the pelvis and helps the baby to get into a good position for birth, *in sha' Allah*. Additionally, walking during labor is said to actually speed the labor and should be encouraged for as long as the mother feels able to remain up and physically <u>Active</u>.

Yoga type stretching builds overall flexibility. Special care should be taken with Yoga and there are specially trained prenatal Yoga instructor certifications for training with expectant mothers. As *Muslims* we must take care to utilize the physical benefits of Yoga, but avoid the erroneous spiritual teachings that may accompany it.

There are a series of well-known exercises designed specifically for our birthing muscles. These focus on strengthening the leg muscles, stretching the birthing muscles, improving lower extremity circulation, and maintaining mother's flexibility to *Actively* give birth.

As with any exercise program, expectant women should start slow and consult their care provider if they have any concerns. Be sure to "listen" to your body and don't overdo it. Exercise should never "hurt" and obviously, while pregnant, should not focus on flattening the abdomen.

I am a firm believer in the simple pregnancy focused exercises that Dr. Bradley taught in his work, none of which are strenuous or aerobic. However, they are great for preparing the muscles and tissues needed for birth. These are best taught in a class setting to ensure understanding and proper form. Susan McCutcheon's book, <u>Natural Childbirth the Bradley Way</u> has good illustrations of these exercises, however be forewarned there are quite a few naked photos in her book.

- <u>Crisscross Floor Sitting</u> – sitting cross-legged on the floor (like school children, called "Indian-Style" when I was a child, called "Crisscross-Applesauce" by my children) - This helps to stretch the inner thighs and encourages good circulation to the legs. The mother can also lift her belly up and lean forward (in essence, placing her unborn baby in her lap) to stretch the lower back and relieve pressure from carrying the heavy load, *in sha' Allah*. This also helps to stretch the round ligaments that connect the uterus to the spine. These ligaments will need to stretch during labor as contractions pulls the uterus upwards and outwards. Having prepared these ligaments ahead of time should make the labor a little smoother, *in sha'Allah*.

- Hip Tucks or Pelvic Rocks – this Yoga-type movement gets mother on all fours (hands and knees) as she rocks her hips, first sagging her lower back, then straightening it, then tucking the hips under (she should feel her baby pull up as she tucks) – I find most women have difficulty mastering this at first. We tend to want to hump our upper back or use our shoulders, but this is strictly an exercise of hip movement. When done correctly, this exercise feels great as it provides such relief for aching backs. It also allows our womb to move forward, as it does during labor contractions, and gives the baby extra room to maneuver into a good position, *in sha' Allah*. Doing a generous number of these daily also helps to prepare the uterine muscles for its work at moving forward during labor contractions.

- Squatting – It's important to squat often, keeping your feet flat on the floor (this can be done with a partner for added balance) – Squatting is the naturally ergonomic birthing position for humans. It also opens the outlet of the pelvis by 10% or more, as compared to the standing position, making it easier for the baby to pass into the world, *in sha' Allah*. If we compare squatting to lying on our back, which actually closes pelvic capacity, there is approximately 30%, or more, greater capacity in the pelvic outlet while squatting. This exercise not only flexes your pelvic outlet, it builds strength and stamina in your legs and stretches the perineum (tissues between the vagina and anus which must stretch during the birth).

- Butterfly – this exercise is best done with a partner. The expectant mother sits on the floor, similar to the crisscross position except she should touch the soles of her feet to one another. She should rest her upper back against a support (couch or wall for example) with a 6 to 8 inch gap between her lower back and the support (this slightly leaning back slant allows room for her growing abdomen as she does the exercises). Once in position, her partner sits in front of her and places his/her hands, palms up, under her knees to provide resistance as she presses down towards the floor against him/her. The partner should release the resistance as she raises her knees back up and should not push or force her legs up.

The resistance provided should be enough to give her a bit of a work out without actually stopping her from pressing down.

Kegel (may be the most important of all) - this refers to the group of muscles that stretch from the front to back under your pubic bone. It lies under the perineum, the smooth tissues between the vagina and anus.

Good tone in this muscle group is imperative as baby passes through them. A sagging or poor tone will cause the baby to drag, rather than pass through smoothly. In addition to supporting the weight of your growing baby, these muscles support all of your internal organs and are also called the "pelvic floor muscles."

You should learn to do Kegel exercises now and continue doing them for life. They are known for preventing or helping to heal hemorrhoids, preventing or curing incontinence (peeing yourself when you cough, laugh, or sneeze, which is common in pregnancy and later life for women who have poor Kegel tone) and more, *in sha' Allah*. The good news is that they respond fairly quickly to exercise, *alhamdulillah*.

To find the muscles, simply stop the flow of urine the next time you go to the bathroom; the muscles you use to stop the flow are the muscles I'm talking about. Incidentally, these are also your pushing muscles for birth. Never do Kegel exercises on a full bladder, as you could cause a bladder infection by squeezing urine back up to the bladder. When you're sure you know the muscles, begin simply contracting them (it will feel as if you're pulling everything upward) and work your way up to doing 200 of these daily (think of it as ten sets of twenty).

When the muscle group is strong you can begin to do more complex exercises where you squeeze...then squeeze a little deeper...then a little more (like taking it up the stairs), then hold for 3 seconds, then release down the same 3 steps.

During birth you will push with these muscle and also "let go" with them, as they must be relaxed in order for the baby to pass. Being aware of these muscles and having good tone is one of the most important things you can do to prepare your "bottom area" for birth, *in sha' Allah*.

As briefly stated earlier, in Chapter Eight, if the tone of the Kegel muscle is tight and taut, the birth will be easier. This is because when the baby comes to the pelvic floor it will hit resistance from the tone muscles. The resistance will give in the baby's neck and cause it to flex so that he or she will be born with its chin on its chest, *in sha' Allah*. This ensures that the smallest part of the baby's head is born first and <u>Assists</u> the gentlest stretching of the mother's tissues. It also avoids the baby's neck being hyperflexed backwards, as happens when the baby's face comes out first, rather than the crown of the head.

For more on the importance of the Kegel exercise, I have included an article from my Saudi Life Motherhood column, "Lifelong Pregnancy Exercise":

Lifelong Pregnancy Exercise

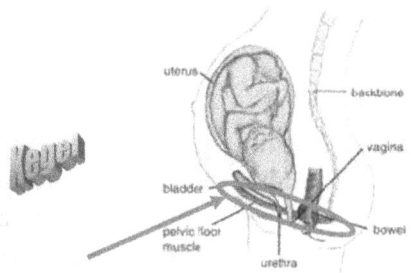

THERE are many exercises designed to prepare women for birth. One of the top ten is squatting. But perhaps even more important is the one that focuses on the rarely discussed muscle that extends from the pubic bone in the front to the tailbone in the back. This muscle is like a sling which supports all of the internal organs and while pregnant, the baby. During birth the baby must pass through this muscle to be born. Men also have this muscle and it is important for both genders to maintain its tone lifelong.

It is often called the pelvic floor muscle or the Kegel muscle, after Dr. Arnold Kegel who discovered it in the late 1940s. Dr. Kegel also discovered the importance of exercising this muscle for good tone.

A weak Kegel muscle will result in incontinence (leaking urine, especially when coughing, sneezing, or laughing), hemorrhoids, uterine prolapse (the womb actually falls out of the woman's body), or prostate cancer in men. When the muscle is in poor tone during birth the baby will drag the muscle rather than smoothly pass through it.

The good news is that it responds rather quickly to exercise. The exercises to tone the muscle are called Kegels. When the muscle is tone it will help prevent hemorrhoids or help heal existing ones. It will also cause the baby's chin to press down against baby's chest during birth which results in the smallest part of the baby's head being born first, meaning less likelihood for tears or need for stitches after birth.

To find the muscle simply stop the flow of urine while using the toilet. The muscle squeezed to control the flow is the Kegel muscle. This is the same muscle used to excrete bowel movements and to push the baby out at birth. It should be noted that the Kegel muscle should not be exercised on a full bladder as it could cause bladder infection.

During Bradley Method® classes we start by having mothers and fathers learn to recognize the muscle and simply squeeze and let the tightness fade away. We encourage doing five sets of ten squeezes daily (fifty).

Over the course of twelve weeks we teach progressively complicated toning exercises until they are contracting the muscle tighter, up three levels and then releasing with control back down three levels. By the end of the class our students are doing two hundred daily.

A tone Kegel muscle is one of the best-kept secrets to better birth as well as sexual health and control. It should be one taught early in life and continued into old age.

I also advocate for hip rotations, which can be done with or without the aid of a birth ball. This exercise simply involves the mother rotating her hips, while in a sitting position, in wide circles to increase flexibility and range of motion, which aids in assuming various labor and birth positions.

The key is to keep your body healthy, fit, flexible, and _Active_ for the best possible birthing conditions for you, _in sha' Allah_. The design of birth is as perfect as the Creator; however, it is up to us to maximize that design by ensuring we tie our camels in preparation for the event.

CHAPTER 15

Birth Consumerism

Your preparation for your birth will play a big role in your birth experience, *in sha' Allah*. However, enough cannot be said about the influence and power that your birth attendant(s) and birthplace have over you and your experience. Once you are in labor, it's very difficult to shop around for the right caregiver to support you during your birth. I cannot sufficiently stress the importance of choosing your birth team and birthplace wisely. Much thought and effort should go into this critical decision and it should never be made lightly.

Consider your first few prenatal visits a time to interview the provider as a potential birth attendant. Don't fall into a mindset of being "stuck" with a doctor or birthplace, simply because you've started a file with them. The earlier you do this the better. However, it's never too late in your pregnancy to shop around; that is, until the labor starts!

Find out the care provider's education as well as experience with, and feelings about, the type of birth you hope to have. You might be surprised to realize that many obstetric doctors and nurses have never seen (or rarely ever see) a completely natural birth. The exposure and trust in truly natural birth simply isn't taught in medical school.

If you are in an area that is served by midwives, count your blessings and take advantage of the opportunity to birth with one! The midwifery model of care is founded on family education and is typically far more mother-focused than the obstetric counterpart. However, just because she is a midwife doesn't remove your responsibility to ask questions and get a feel for her philosophies to ensure they gel with yours.

An example of the importance of being an *Active* birth consumer is in consideration of episiotomy. This is a surgical incision in the mother's genital region to make the birth canal larger that some care providers insist is "necessary" in order for the baby to come out. Chapter 11 included an article from my Saudi Life Motherhood column, "Many Mothers Routinely "Cut" at Delivery." If you get a chance to read it online, be sure to scan the comments for testimonials of many mothers who have birthed without this procedure, which too many physicians continue to perform as a matter of barbaric routine, despite the evidence against this practice.

In fact, in the AMANI Birth philosophy it is clear from the get go that the parents truly have the most *Active* role in the care of their unborn child. To understand the mother's duty to take an *Active* part in her own care, I have included two articles from my Saudi Life Motherhood column, "Pregnancy Primary Care Provider" and "Shopping for a Doctor."

Pregnancy Primary Care Provider

MY personal experience with care during pregnancy, labor, and birth are set in the context of the obstetric models of the United States, Egypt, and Saudi Arabia. Because of their systems of medically dominant maternity services, I automatically associate *Primary Care Provider* for pregnancy with "*Obstetrician.*"

In fact, it wasn't until I started getting more involved in the global natural birth movement that I realized that in much of the developed world Midwives fulfill this role, with statistically better outcomes (Wagner, 2008).

Then I started to consider, who acts as a *Primary Care Provider* and what is their role in pregnancy and birth? When I looked it up I found the following definition:

primary care provider - *a person who helps in identifying or preventing or treating illness or disability* (Farlex, Inc., 2011)

In the context of pregnancy, labor, and birth, I am uncomfortable with categorizing these very normal life events in the same group as illness and disability. So I kept searching. Next, I found an article that had a definition that started me thinking:

"A primary care provider is the 'captain' of a team...who care for the same patient." (Mueller, 2009).

But then again, there's the word *patient* that I really don't identify with either. In fact, when I stop to consider the implications, I come to the conclusion that the woman should be the *'captain'* of her team and truly is her own *primary care provider* during her pregnancy, labor, and birth; or at least she should be.

From my perspective, she isn't a *passive patient* to be treated; she is an *Active* participant who is venturing on a journey in the natural cycle of life (Balaskas, 1992). In fact, it is the woman who has ultimate control of her body and thus the care of her pregnancy and her baby. Only she determines which nutrients, vitamins, or medications she puts into her pregnancy and her baby. Only she controls her state of physical preparedness for the big event of birth. Nutrition and exercise are the two variables that we have true control over. Frankly, they may be the most important factors determining the safe range of options open to her and they will have the greatest affect on the short and long term outcomes for mother and child.

It is the woman who ultimately decides how well she will take care of herself each day during her pregnancy. She is the one who decides whether or not to educate herself in order to make informed decisions about her care. She decides who to give her trust to and whose advice she will follow throughout her journey to motherhood.

No one can force a test or procedure or intervention on her until she walks out her front door and turns her control over. She has the right and responsibility to know her options, seek information, and make decisions about what will or will not be done to her or her baby. There are many different types of childbirth 'experts' and 'philosophies' and her baby is counting on her to sort through it all in order to act in his/her best interest.

The same is true for the care of her child as he/she grows. It will be the parents, primarily the mother, who will decided when to seek outside intervention of care at every step along the path to adulthood. She will decide when an illness can be nurtured at home or if it should be elevated to medicinal intervention. She will act or not by staying home with her child or venturing out to the clinic or hospital to invite 'expert' medical care for him/her for many years to come.

This means that primary care begins at home and doesn't end until her death and, in the case of her child, at the age of his/her own adult consent. With this in mind, women need to wake up to the reality that both mother's and baby's health hang in the balance of the big and little decisions she makes during pregnancy, birth, and beyond.

Each one of us is ultimately responsible for all of the choices we make and it's time we focus on the consequences and heed the global call of Midwife, Lonnie Morris when she says, "Women of Earth, take back your birth!" Thinking in terms of who's your primary care provider, I couldn't say it better myself!

Shopping for a Doctor

DURING a recent childbirth class my students asked me to write about shopping for a maternity care provider. They were a bit perplexed by the idea of shopping around or interviewing for the right doctor (or midwife). It seems most expectant parents are more aware of the idea of shopping for the "best" hospital and then just accepting the doctors that are there.

With this mentality they really miss the point of being a good birth consumer. It's important to recognize that it is the doctor/midwife, not the hospital that will most determine the atmosphere and outcome of your birth experience. You must find someone that you feel comfortable trusting during one of the most vulnerable times in your lives.

Below are some questions to contemplate when considering a care provider. Be sure to ask open ended, nonleading questions to elicit their true stance on issues.

What routine procedures do you typically follow during labor and birth?

1. Are you open to exceptions?
2. Why would you suggest an induction?
3. What is your induction rate (an educated guess is good enough)?
4. Under what circumstance would you recommend a cesarean?
5. What is your cesarean rate (an educated guess is good enough)?
6. How often do you perform episiotomy?
7. What measures would you take to support the perineum without cutting?
8. How do you feel about intermittent fetal monitoring with non-ultrasound device (periodically using a fetal stethoscope instead of a continuous electric fetal monitor or periodic handheld Doppler)?
9. How would you feel attending a birth with no interventions (no IV, no vaginal exams, no drugs to speed labor, no pain medications, no breaking of waters, no cutting)?
10. What positions would you feel comfortable allowing for the birth?
11. How long are you willing to wait before clamping the umbilical cord?
12. Would you allow more than one companion in for the labor and/or birth?
13. If I need cesarean, will my companion(s) be allowed to accompany me?
14. How do you feel about breast versus bottle-feeding?
15. How many natural births have you attended (clarify no drugs used during labor or birth)?

It's important to get a sense for the person's feelings in regards to things that are important to you. Your list of questions may look different based on what you want for your birth. Watch their body language and facial expressions as they respond.

If the doctor will not even entertain your questions, cut your losses and move on. The same goes if they are patronizing in their responses. If they criticize openly or through body language and/or facial expressions, do not expect many concessions when the birth comes.

However, if they seem interested in your birth plan and even willing to know more about why you want such an experience, there is hope. Are they willing to review the evidence with you on topics which they may be unfamiliar (such as current recommendations regarding upright positions for birth, delayed cord clamping, or birth without episiotomy)?

The bottom line is that you choose them and it should be you who makes the decisions regarding what happens in all nonemergency situations. If you don't feel supported, you probably aren't. Tune into your intuition. Don't wait until it's time to push to decide you chose the wrong provider

CHAPTER 16

Freedom of Movement and Birth Positions

One of the most important things a mother can do to work with her body during labor and cope with the discomforts is to stay *Active* throughout the event. It is imperative that she be encouraged to walk for as long as she is able and that she be allowed freedom to move and try different positions.

The mother who remains *Active* and purposeful in her movements will be in much better control of herself and will be able to significantly reduce her discomfort while improving the birth experience and shortening the length of labor, *in sha' Allah*. Besides walking, she may also find rocking, swaying her hips, or assuming various positions and purposefully experimenting with whatever movements that come naturally to her to be soothing and comforting during her labor. These movements also assist in the mother-baby dance and may encourage the baby to assume the best position for birth and ease his/her movements through the mother's pelvis.

First Stage Labor

As discussed in Chapter Nine, first stage labor is divided into three parts: Early, *Active*, and Transition. During the early phase, the contractions are typically nothing more than a distraction. At this point it's best if she doesn't pay too much attention to them. Positions for this stage are simply associated with the activity of the moment. If it's middle of the night, she should relax and rest, as it may fizzle out and stop or it may go on for quite some time and she'll need her energy later. If she's hungry she should eat, as she won't be able to eat much later and she'll need all the fuel she can get. If she's wide-awake and full of energy she might consider going for a walk. As noted before, walking will help to open the inlet of the pelvis and is said to speed the labor, and at very least it will keep her from focusing on it too soon. In fact, in randomized trials, walking during labor results not only in potentially shorter labors, but also seems to reduce the need for pain medication, reduces the incidence of fetal heart abnormalities, and lessens the likelihood for oxytocic drugs that are often used to speed labor.

When she gets to hard or _Active_ labor, she may be able to continue in _Active_, upright positions for quite some time. She may still walk between contractions, rock her hips on a birth ball, find relief in pelvic rocking movements on her hands and knees between contractions, or assume any other position that helps her to find comfort and ease. However, at some point she will most likely need to lie down. By then her contractions are probably hard and well established and may be coming one right after the next. For this strong and hard labor she will likely find the most relief in complete relaxation. It is best if she has practiced deep relaxation during her pregnancy to really master what works for her and to recognize the difference between partial and complete relaxing of muscles. At this time, the more she tenses any area of her body during a contraction, the more intense her pains will be.

The good news is that she has control over unnecessary pain that comes from fighting her labor. She can minimize how much she hurts by assuming positions that maximize the forces of gravity and work with her body during labor. She can also reduce the amount of pain she experiences by surrendering herself to the labor and allowing her body to do its work. This comes back to completely relaxing every muscle in her body so that all of the energy and blood flow is concentrated in her womb as it automatically does its job.

Relaxation Position

Typically, a side-lying position that allows the abdomen to fall forward towards the bed is most conducive to maximizing the force of gravity. Realizing that the uterus moves forward during each contraction and facilitating this with her forward falling abdomen will ensure that her position is most conducive to what's naturally occurring in her body. The medical term for the described side-lying position is the Sims' position (shown below). Notice that the bottom arm is behind her, not under her body or her head. Also note that the bottom leg is also back, with the top leg forward. Typically you would slant a pillow under her head and upper shoulder so that it supports the head, top shoulder, top arm and hand. Be sure that the pillow is not wedged under the lower shoulder, as this would be uncomfortable. A second pillow would be placed under her knee, lower leg, ankle, and foot of the top leg for support. In this way no part of her body is stressing on any other. Most mothers find this ergonomic position to be conducive to restful sleep in the later months of pregnancy, as well as the most relaxing position during hard labor. This position is one that the AMANI Birth Instructor will ensure mothers are well acquainted with.

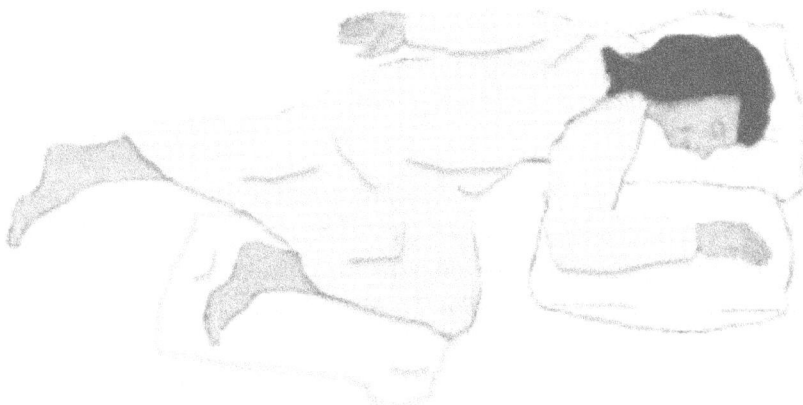

Sims' or Side-Lying Relaxation Position

On thing to note is that the circulation is best when the mother lies on her left side. Although the Prophet (*Sallallaahu 'alayhi wa sallam*) taught us to lie on our right, it is not *haram* (sin) to lay on the left. In the case of pregnancy, the physiology supports a left side position and most women find it very uncomfortable to lay any other way, no matter how desperately they'd like to turn over.

For more about left side laying positions, I've included an article from my Saudi Life Motherhood column, "Pregnancy Sleep Positions in the News."

Pregnancy Sleep Positions in the News

WITH each of my pregnancies I found it near impossible to be comfortable sleeping in any position other than my left side. I even have some distant recollection of reading "something, somewhere" that stated that there can be restricted blood flow when laying on the right side due to the weight of the baby, thus making it better to sleep on the left side.

However, these vague references and personal experience aren't really enough to start a pregnancy sleeping campaign. Even so, when I teach relaxation and discuss positions with pregnant women I advise them to lay mostly on their left sides due this "something" that is compressed under the weight of the baby, therefore making it "better" to lay on the left.

As a *Muslimah*, this poses some dilemma, as I know there are *hadeeths* of the Prophet (*Sallallaahu 'alayhi wa sallam*) recommending we sleep on our right sides.

Narrated Al-Bara' bin 'Azib: When Allah's Apostle went to bed, he used to sleep on his right side and then say, "All-ahumma aslamtu nafsi ilaika, wa wajjahtu wajhi ilaika, wa fauwadtu Amri ilaika, wa alja'tu zahri ilaika, raghbatan warahbatan ilaika. La Malja'a wa la manja minka illa ilaika. Amantu bikitabika al-ladhi anzalta wa nabiyyika al-ladhi arsalta." Allah's Apostle said, "Whoever recites these words (before going to bed) and dies the same night, he will die on the Islamic religion (as a Muslim)."

Narrated Al-Bara 'bin 'Azib: The Prophet said: "Whenever you go to bed perform ablution like that for the prayer, lie or your right side and say, "Allahumma aslamtu wajhi ilaika, wa fauwadtu amri ilaika, wa alja'tu Zahri ilaika raghbatan wa rahbatan ilaika. La Malja' wa la manja minka illa ilaika. Allahumma amantu bikitabika-l-ladhi anzalta wa bina-biyika-l ladhi arsalta" (O Allah! I surrender to You and entrust all my affairs to You and depend upon You for Your Blessings both with hope and fear of You. There is no fleeing from You, and there is no place of protection and safety except with You O Allah! I believe in Your Book (the Qur'an) which You have revealed and in Your Prophet (Muhammad) whom You have sent). Then if you die on that very night, you will die with faith (i.e. or the religion of Islam). Let the aforesaid words be your last utterance (before sleep)." I repeated it before the Prophet and when I reached "Allahumma amantu bikitabika-l-ladhi anzalta (O Allah I believe in Your Book which You have revealed)." I said, "Wa-rasulika (and your Apostle)." The Prophet said, "No, (but say): 'Wanabiyika-l-ladhi arsalta (Your Prophet whom You have sent), instead."

In the News

This week the news is abuzz about a report out of The University of Auckland in New Zealand about a suspicious link between sleeping on the back and right side during late pregnancy and incidence of stillbirth. Association between maternal sleep practices and risk of late stillbirth: a case-control study Surprisingly, it even made the local news in Arabic.

It's important to note that the report does not profess to make a direct link between mothers' sleep positions and stillbirth. It clearly states:

"This is the first study to report maternal sleep related practices as risk factors for stillbirth, and these findings require urgent confirmation in further studies."

"Our findings might be due to restricted blood flow to the baby which can occur when the mother lies on her back or right side for long periods. If confirmed through future studies we may be able to reduce the number of stillbirths by up to a third, which is incredibly exciting. We are now trying to obtain funding to conduct this further research."

"Further research is needed as a matter of urgency so that pregnant women can receive the best public health advice about sleep position."

Obviously, it is just a beginning of needed research. However, it does show a logic behind my personal experiences and gives some credibility to my advice to expectant mothers, *alhamdulillah*.

On the other hand, it still leaves me perplexed with the recommendation in the *hadith*. I turned to my husband for some guidance in this regard and he said:

Sleeping on the right side is *Sunnah*, not *fardh* (obligatory)

Sleeping on the left side is permissible and not *haram* (sin)

The Prophet (peace be upon him) was referring to normal circumstances, not pregnancy

My conclusion is that it makes sense that the Prophet (*Sallallaahu 'alayhi wa sallam*) would have excused someone with a broken arm or burn or the like on his right side. Similarly, since there is evidence to suggest that the mother's and baby's circulation can be compromised by the weight of the baby while lying on her back or right side that left side lying may be the logical choice during pregnancy.

Sleeping positions during pregnancy for mothers' and babies' health and let the evidence be clear so there is no illusion of sleeping against the Prophet's (peace be upon him) advice.

Deep Relaxation

To reach a level of truly deep relaxation, she should begin by keeping her eyes closed, jaw relaxed, mouth open, and relax even the tongue in her mouth. She should aim for the deep sleep relaxation that leads to drooling on the pillow. By keeping her mouth open she will facilitate the softening and opening of the tissues of the birth canal. In the words of world-renowned midwife, author, and lecture, Ina May Gaskin, "An open jaw is an open vagina."

Next, she should ensure that her neck, shoulders, arms, and hands are loose and limp. She should keep her hands open and avoid clenching her fists. Even slight tension in her smallest finger may intensify the abdominal tightening she experiences with contractions. Moving the focus downwards, she should ensure that the voluntary abdominal and back muscles are completely relaxed, the sphincter muscles of the urethra, vagina, and anus are loose, and the hips and buttocks are also completely relaxed. The same goes down her legs from her thigh to her calves to her feet and her toes.

This is an excellent time for her labor companion or coach to get involved and assess her position and relaxation. Ideally, he or she should have practiced this with her in the weeks and months leading up to the birth. The companion should be astute at recognizing her tensions and encouraging her to let go. A soft touch and gentle reminder to relax each of the aforementioned areas of her body will go a long way in helping her release unconscious tension that may cause increased pain with each contraction.

Additionally, she should maintain normal breathing that is deep and cleansing. She should not pant or chest breath in labor. Each breath should result in the rise and fall of her abdomen. Her companion should encourage her to bring her breathing deeper and deeper with each breath. Breathing in rhythm with her and encouraging her to breath slowly and calmly will help her to relax even more, *in sha' Allah*. Taking one contraction at a time, in a relaxed and calm manner will facilitate the ease with which her body can effectively work to open for her baby.

Transition

As she reaches the end of first stage, her womb will transition to full dilation and the contractions will shift gears from those that work to open her tissues, to those that provide a strong downward force to push the baby out. Transition is a time of change in the pattern of her labor. She usually will not recognize what is happening physically but may have a strong emotional reaction to the different sensations during this time. Many mothers become confused, upset, angry, frustrated, defeated, and scared at this time. She may say things like, "**I can't do this anymore**," "**I give up**," "**I hate you!**" "**Just give me the drugs!**" "**I can't take the pain**," etc. This is understandable as her body is performing a function that is foreign to her and it causes a sense of self-doubt and upset, along with discomfort and pain.

The good news is that the transition stage, although it can be quite traumatic, doesn't last long. A good labor companion has been clued up on what emotional signs to expect and can recognize it for what it is. With a lot of verbal encouragement, eye contact, and guidance, the companion can help her through, one contraction at a time. If she can manage through one contraction, then the next, she is well on her way to the birth of her baby. Typically the emotional turmoil of this stage only persists for 10 to 30 minutes.

Remember the deep relaxation techniques described for the hard labor of first stage, coupled with calm, deep abdominal breathing. These tools will help minimize her discomfort and get her through. As second stage approaches, her contractions will space out, giving her more rest time between sensations, which will allow her to recoup her energy and get to the business of birthing her baby, *in sha' Allah*.

Second Stage Labor

Interestingly, when you observe the customs and practices of current generations of hospital birthers, you will find a great deal of them on their back with their feet up in stirrups to deliver. As noted in Chapter One, this custom came about when a medical doctor became obsessed with observing births after the death of his own young sister and her unborn child due to labor complications in the 1600s. Of course, if a woman has submitted herself to epidural, it's an understandable position, albeit the worst physiological position for birth, since her legs are likely to be floppy and paralyzed and she can't really assume any other position. On her back and in stirrups truly makes the birth of the baby harder than it needs to be. Mothers should be encouraged to persevere through labor without medicinal pain relief to avoid the many complications that come with being stuck on her back for delivery, the most problematic of all positions.

In fact, if you view any ancient artifacts or drawings of women birthing you will notice that they are usually depicted in a squatting position. Moreover, if left to their own instincts, no woman in her right mind would throw herself onto her back and lift her legs in the air at the moment of birth. It frankly just doesn't make sense!

Taking a closer look at how your body works in labor and birth, it's easy to see why lying on your back is the worst possible position for any pregnant, let alone laboring or birthing, woman.

First of all, there are major blood vessels that run up and down the spine. With the added weight of the baby there is a risk of slowing the blood flow, which can result in less oxygenation for both mother and baby. This condition can alter the mother's blood pressure and cause her to lose the stamina needed to experience a completely natural birth. Additionally, this lack of oxygenation can cause the baby to suffer from "fetal distress," which is one of the most common reasons cited for emergency cesarean delivery.

Digging a bit further we come to realize that lying on our back also fights gravity, which requires the muscles of the womb to work harder than they should have to in order to eject the baby. This is two faceted. First of all, consider that the baby should be coming down through the mother's pelvis and out through her birth canal. However, when she lies on her back, the pelvis and birth canal are no longer "down," but instead the path of birth is horizontal, requiring much more muscular force than upright positions.

Additionally, as mentioned before, the movement of the womb during contractions is a forward movement that pulls the baby somewhat forward, out in front of the mother's abdomen. This forward movement helps to get the baby in alignment for the journey into the world. If a woman is in an upright, and especially slightly forward-leaning position, she puts gravity to work with her womb, reducing the muscular efforts needed to move the womb forward. Contrarily, laying on the back works against gravity, as the womb has to work much harder to move forward when the whole weight of the baby is now pulling it back towards her spine. **Simply put lying on your back fights the natural force of gravity and makes labor and birth harder, longer, and more painful.**

Being on our back may make us good and complacent patients of our doctors, but it does not make sense in birth. Another profound issue is the size of the outlet of the pelvis. When we assume a squatting position, the outlet of our pelvis opens and increases in diameter by about 10% or more, as compared to standing or other upright positions. But worse than this is the fact that lying on our back actually closes off the pelvic outlet, and even more so when our legs are raised in the air, as is the case with the use of stirrups. It's estimated that the difference in the circumference of the pelvic outlet is about 30%, when we compare lying on our back with our feet up to a complete squat. This can be a substantial difference, especially for large size babies.

Clearly, with all that's been said here, it's obvious to conclude that the squatting position is the most effective for birthing a baby. Additionally, the squatting position shortens the birth canal, which also adds to its efficiency in the birth process. However, not all women have the stamina to squat, or a birthing stool or supportive assistant to help them maintain this position for the length of time it may take to complete the pushing phase of labor. It's a good idea to be familiar with a variety of positions and alternate them in cases of a long or difficult second stage (pushing stage).

Common alternative positions can include side-lying, hands-and-knees, semi-sitting (only marginally better than lying on the back), asymmetrical with one leg up and the other down, etc. A woman should be free to change positions between contractions and encouraged to assume the position that feels best to her. It should be the honor and duty of the care provider to respect the woman's choice and adjust himself or herself to her position, rather than dominating her position for their own convenience.

As birthing women in a normal, natural case scenario, it is important that we tune into our bodies and advocate for ourselves to avoid being coerced into birthing situations that go against our natural instinct to be an Active participant in the birth of our baby, rather than a submissive patient undergoing a medical procedure. It truly is time to head the common mantra stated before, "Women of Earth, take back your birth!"

CHAPTER 17

Minimizing and Coping With Pain

At some point during the labor the mother is likely to move from a perception of labor "discomfort" to labor "pain." Some mothers will reach this threshold earlier than others. Fortunate are the mothers who keep the perspective that labor is a positive surge of energy and never relate the sensations of labor with "pain." Regardless of how you describe or relate to the sensations, maintaining a positive attitude about the experience is still a key factor in coping with pain. Understanding that the process of labor has a purpose makes it easier to tolerate. Also remember that *Allah* will not burden us with more than we can bear.

> *"We do not burden any human being with more than he is well able to bear..."* [Qur'an 23:62]

Additionally, the physical considerations from Chapter 16 will significantly reduce unnecessary pain and also allow her to cope with the discomfort she does experience. When the labor becomes strong and overwhelming, a mother who assumes an ergonomic position that works with the natural process and employs techniques for complete relaxation of all muscles groups will experience far less pain than the mother who tightens up or fights her labor.

With this in mind, it is important that a laboring mother not tighten up even the most insignificant of muscles. Any tension she holds in her body has the potential to increase the sensations of pain. Her labor companions should carefully observe her for any tense muscles and encourage her to completely let go and relax. She should remain still during the hardest part of labor in deep concentration on relaxing every single muscle. Her forehead should be relaxed, eyes closed, jaw relaxed, mouth open, and even the tongue in her mouth relaxed. In fact, deep relaxation that results in drooling on the pillow is what she's after.

Massage and Touch

Her labor companions can help her remember these points, as well as massage or stroke the tension out of her shoulders, hips, legs and feet. They can also ensure her hands are open and relaxed. Providing counter pressure against an aching lower back or tailbone, or gently squeezing the hips together can also provide much relief. Follow her cues, but never stop what you're doing in the middle of a contraction unless she indicates to do so. She probably won't be able to acknowledge or confirm that she likes what you are doing, but if you stop it can totally throw her off, causing unnecessary panic or pain.

Forward Positions

Remember that her position should assist the uterus as it moves forward during contractions. Any position that facilitates this forward-falling action will reduce the amount of effort the uterine muscles must exert, and thus make her labor more effective, quicker, and less painful, *in sha' Allah*. Be sure to master the side-lying position discussed in Chapter 16.

Don't Imitate Media Births

Unfortunately, rapid chest breathing and panting, as is often depicted in television or movie dramatizations of birth, is likely to cause tension, panic, fear, and more pain. Women who have not prepared for their birth and only have these media visions of birth are apt to employ these potentially dangerous breathing patterns. What's worse, well-intending hospital staff may even recommend them.

The trouble with chest breathing is that it alters the oxygen and carbon dioxide mix in the blood, resulting in inadequate oxygenation for both mother and baby. Conversely, breathing in a calm and deep manner will assist the mother in maintaining a totally relaxed posture while providing adequate oxygenation to her baby. In fact, simply remembering to breath in natural, deep breaths may avert bouts of fetal distress. The deep breaths of a calm, confident mother in labor will exude peace and permit her to surrender to the birth experience, *in sha' Allah*.

Surrender

Moreover, surrendering to the labor experience is an important part of the journey to motherhood. The sooner she can emotionally and physically let go and let birth happen, the better. She is much more likely to do this in an atmosphere of loving trust and support, than in a rushed and harried environment of urgency.

Surrender is also an important component of trusting *Allah* during this vulnerable time. Surrendering to her labor is an act of worship by surrendering to *Allah*, the Creator of the amazing process of birth.

The Companion's Role

The labor companions can be of great support during the hardest parts of labor. Simply being a supportive force that believes in the woman and trusts *Allah's* design will enable her to go on through her journey with greater ease. Things that can specifically be done include:

1. Encourage her to let go and surrender to *Allah* and make *dua*.

2. Remind her to breathe calmly and deeply.

3. Breathe with her and guide her breaths deeper and deeper as she relaxes.

4. Encourage her to close her eyes or look into her eyes if she insists on keeping them open, as eye contact can go a long way towards combating fear.

5. Express your trust in *Allah* and faith in her ability to do this.

6. Help her focus on just one contraction at a time. One by one, you will get through this.

7. Remind her to relax and loosen every part of her body, starting from her forehead, to her jaw and tongue in the mouth, across her neck and shoulders, down her arms, through her abdomen, and down her hips and legs, all the way to her toes.

8. Massage her body and apply pressure in ways that relax and alleviate pain (keep in tune with her and try counter pressure on her lower back, squeezing her hips together, pressing against her knees while she is in a sitting position with her back supported against a solid surface).

9. Don't stop whatever you are doing during her contractions unless she tells you to. If you are talking, keep talking, if you are massaging, keep massaging, etc. If you are touching her in any way and notice a tense part of her body you want to address with stroking or massage, do not remove your hands abruptly from her body; instead, walk your hands up or down her body without losing contact so that she doesn't panic wondering where you went, even for a second.

10. Do not ask her questions during contractions or cause her to lose her focus to answer you (she will let you know, probably abruptly, if she doesn't like the way you are touching her during the contraction, don't doubt yourself, keep doing what you're doing, and ask her between contractions if you are unsure).

11. Giver her permission to make noise and encourage her to get her *hassanat* (rewards) by calling out to *Allah* as she vocalizes.

12. Help her to change positions between contractions if she'd like and encourage her to drink water, eat a small amount of dates, and purge her bladder and bowels often. Wipe her forehead with a cool cloth and offer anything she needs.

To a great extent, she really does have control over how much the labor sensations hurt. Combining a positive attitude with physical ergonomics, relaxation, and a sense of emotional security will go a long way in easing her discomfort and empowering her to experience the miracle of giving birth that leaves her feeling extremely euphoric as she bonds with her baby, *in sha' Allah*.

CHAPTER 18

What to Expect in <u>AMANI</u> Birth Training-Part Three

The *Active* Series focuses on staying healthy and preparing your body during pregnancy and remaining a cognizant, aware participant during the labor so that the mother can give birth to her baby, rather than be delivered of it. Remaining in control of her body by staying off medicinal pain medications will allow her to keep *Active* and mobile for as long as she can. Once her ability to walk and remain upright becomes impeded by the progressing labor, she should still remain *Active* in employing labor and birth positions that are most conducive to the task at hand.

Understanding how your body works in labor and birth will help you to assist the natural forces that automatically take over during this time. Unfortunately, too many women face their labor without this understanding and inadvertently fight the process and make things far harder on themselves than they need to be. The key in this series is to discover the best techniques to remain an *Active* giver of birth, *in sha' Allah*.

The *Active* series is compiled of four modules:

Module 1   Pregnancy Exercise

In this module we will focus on the importance of remaining physically active during pregnancy. It will also explore the many exercises that are especially designed to develop the strength and stamina that will be needed during labor and birth. Many of the exercises are aimed at stretching and increasing flexibility of the tissues and muscles that will be most effected and needed during the birth process. None of the pregnancy exercises are strenuous and your AMANI Birth Teacher will demonstrate and ensure you are able to do them all.

Module 2   Pregnancy Nutrition

This module will demonstrate the importance that daily nutrition plays in the final outcomes for both mother and baby. Every day and each meal are vital to the best health and welfare of the baby. Understanding that the baby is developing rapidly and at prescribed times illustrates the fact that there is no time when skimping on nutrition is acceptable. There are no "re-do's" in the growth and development of your child in the womb. Thankfully, nutrition is the one thing that the mother has the most control of during her pregnancy. She can make a difference in the health of her child as well as influence her own labor experience, simply by being healthy and well fed.

Module 3   Birthing Positions

This module will explore the evolving history of birthing positions versus the instinctual positions for labor and birth. We will discuss the importance of preparing the body for flexibility and stamina to maintain the most effective birthing positions as well as the need to advocate for this simple right in the medical birthing system. The mother's freedom to remain _Active_ during her labor and encouragement to tune in to her own body to choose the positions that work best for her are a simple matter of human rights.

Module 4   Labor Practice

In this module, the expectant mother and her companion(s) will work to tie together the many pieces of the puzzle as they learn and grow together. They will simulate labor so that by the time the big day arrives, they should function together like the well-trained team that they have become.

It's important that they have not only worked together and practiced labor positions and strategies for natural pain management but that they have communicated these strategies with their birth team. Their birth attendant should be well aware of her plans to remain active during as much of the labor as possible, to utilize deep relaxation and vocalization for the peak of her journey, and to actively participate and utilize a myriad of positions for her birth. No one should be shocked or surprised at her determination to birth naturally and everyone should work together to help her achieve her desired experience.

Part Four - *Natural*

Let us begin with the assumption of normal. What this means is that we enter pregnancy and birth with trust that *Allah* is the Creator of our bodies and HE designed birth as a normal, *Natural* bodily function.

If the mother is healthy and the pregnancy is normal we start out assuming the labor and birth will also be normal. This is far from the current medical model, which trains obstetricians on all of the possible "abnormalities" of pregnancy, labor, and birth to the point that they often see birth as a medical process, rather than the normal, *Natural* life event that it should be.

We can hardly blame doctors for introducing interventions when this is what they are trained to do. We also must remember that each member of our birthing team is an integral part of our birth event. Unfortunately, when those around us are trained to dominate the *Natural* process and revere it with a sense of fear and apprehension, our birth experience will forever be altered into one of debilitating protocols and procedures. Somehow, we must find a way to reserve those interventions for the rare few that truly need it. In fact, the World Health Organization has stated,

"The aim...is to achieve a healthy mother and child with the least possible level of intervention that is compatible with safety. This approach implies that:
...there should be a valid reason to interfere with the *Natural* process."

This means that we really shouldn't be interfering with the *Natural* process of birth as a matter of routine or protocol. Yet, that's exactly what happens in the majority of hospital births.

Remember that birth interventions are relatively new, as the movement of women to the hospitals to deliver began taking place only within the last century. Additionally, if you ponder the longevity and history of human development, both support women in trusting *Allah's* design for the birth process.

CHAPTER 19

Labor Has a Purpose

As believers in *Allah* as the perfect Creator of all things we come to realize that HE didn't arbitrarily sentence mothers to labor. In fact, we trust that our labor has a purpose and *Allah* knows best. It's baffling to hear cases of women electing major abdominal surgery out of their fear of having a *Natural* birth. In fact, *Allah* tells us in the *Qur'an,*

> *"...it may well be that you hate a thing while it is good for you, and it may well be that you love a thing while it is bad for you: and God knows, whereas you do not know. [Qur'an 2:216]*

Although this verse does not specifically refer to labor, I truly feel often applies. Moreover, when we ponder some of the possible reasons for labor we can come up with quite a long list, *subhan'Allah*. In fact, as Jay Hathaway, cofounder of the American Academy of Husband Coached Childbirth® said in an article that is printed in the <u>Bradley Method® Student Workbook,</u>

> *"...there are some very good reasons for labor and they have little,*

if anything to do with cervical dilation."

Let's examine some of the reasons that labor is good for us:

Demand to Take Notice

First of all, it demands our attention and warns us that a major life-changing event is about to happen. This usually allows us time to get to our chosen birthing place, make our nest, and ensure that the people we want to attend to our care and to share this experience are present.

Best Positions

Secondly, if left to follow our _Natural_ urges, it precipitates our movements into positions that are the safest and most conducive to birthing our babies. For example, when I had my youngest daughter, undisturbed at home, I had just entered the washroom between contractions to empty my bladder and bowel. As I stood up I had a contraction that brought me to my knees. I didn't realize at the time that I wouldn't be getting up from this position until I had my baby at my breast, *masha'Allah*.

I don't even want to imagine what may have ensued had I remained upright and just dropped my baby from a standing position on the hard tile floor, head first! This low crouching position ensured that my baby had a safe and gentle entrance without any injury or trauma from a long fall, *alhamdulillah*. It also allowed me just enough time to call out to my husband who barely got to me in time to catch her in his loving hands, *masha'Allah*. I truly would not trade those last intense labor pains for a medicated birth, as it was those uninterrupted discomfort that led to the most absolutely amazing bonding experience that my husband and I shared with our new baby girl.

Emotional Adjustment

Third, there is an emotional and spiritual journey to motherhood that climaxes with the labor and birth of the child. I, for one, am quite content being pregnant, *alhamdulillah*. I love to carry my baby around in my growing womb as I go about my business. During pregnancy, I feel good and I'm in no hurry for labor, because I know it will hurt. Additionally, as a mother of eight, I know that there is no other time when I have as much control or protection over my child than when he or she is inside me. I also know that soon enough I will be busy with the tasks of caring for a completely dependent little person, *masha'Allah*, and much of my other obligations and pursuits will have to slow down, if not be put on hold for a while.

As much as I love my babies and I truly enjoy motherhood, I am quite content to wait and stay in the pregnant state for quite some time. But when the waves of labor strike, I reach a point where I just want to get this birth over with. My labor brings me to a state of submission to *Allah's* will, *alhamdulillah*. During which time I transition from "in no hurry to be a new mommy" to " pleading for HIS mercy to finish the birth so that I can hold and cuddle my newborn."

I truly need the breaking point of labor to ready me for motherhood. I trust that *Allah* (*SWT*), in HIS infinite wisdom, knows exactly what each of us needs and takes us through the trials of labor and life in order to guide us to what is best for us, *subhan'Allah*.

Baby's Benefits

Lastly, we cannot discount the baby's participation in his or her own birth. This is as much an experience and an event for them as it is for the mother. Also consider just a couple of the benefits of labor and *Natural* birth for the baby:

1. Acquisition of probiotics that are result from the passage through the birth canal, which are important for good gut flora. In fact, the Gastrointestinal Society of Canada noted that babies that are born by cesarean lack this benefit for up to six months after birth. Moreover, they stated that vaginally born babies benefit from healthy Lactobacillus bacteria, whereas cesarean born infants pick up Staphylococcus bacteria which is a culprit in the dreaded antibiotic resistant MRSA virus that plagues the modern hospital environment.

2. There is also the effect of the tight passage through the mother's vagina that serve to squeeze the fluid from the lungs, nose and mouth. This is called the Fetal Heimlich Maneuver. This occurs most effectively when the mother has not been subjected to the routine cutting of her tissues (episiotomy). In fact, babies born over an intact perineum typically do not need suctioning to breathe, *subhan'Allah*.

Multiple Factors

When you consider all the factors at play during your labor you begin to realize that *Allah* really does have the best plan for everything.

"...the best of planners is Allah." [Qur'an 8:30]

We really cannot improve upon the _Natural_ process, *subhan'Allah*. We can simply tie our camels to best prepare ourselves for it.

CHAPTER 20

Birth is Inherently Safe

During AMANI Birth classes we learn about the physiology of pregnancy, labor and birth. It's truly amazing to discover the many inherent safety nets *Allah* has designed for birth. The key is to do our part to maximize those safeguards with proper diet, exercise, and prenatal care.

We've already discussed many examples of *Natural* safeties of pregnancy and birth.

Chapter 8 – The loosening and expansion of the mother's pelvis (hips) to make room for the baby to pass. This is facilitated by maternal hormones present towards the end of pregnancy, which loosen joints and cartilage. Of course this contributes to the duck-like waddling that is characteristic of late pregnancy, as well as the clumsiness of the hands as the hormones affect all the joints of the mother's body, *subahan'Allah*. Couple the expanding hips with the baby's head being able to mold and compress as it passes through the birth canal and it's easy to see that birth has been carefully designed, *Allahu Akbar*! Additionally, consider the mother's slowed digestion and blood circulation that allows her blood to pick up more nutrients from the intestines for delivery via the placenta to the baby.

Chapter 11 – The first milk (colostrum) serves as a laxative to clear out the baby's intestines, line and protect the gut, and provides important antibodies to the baby as he/she is first exposed to the world. Breastfeeding also causes contractions after birth that will expel the placenta and clamp down on the open blood vessels left behind to prevent the mother from bleeding to death, *in sha' Allah.*

Chapter 14 - The increased blood volume gained during pregnancy that provides much needed extra oxygen for transport across the placenta to the baby, and also is an allowance for the mother's pending blood loss that will occur after the birth, *subhan'Allah!*

Chapter 19 - The probiotics of the mother's birth canal that ensure healthy gut flora for the baby and the Fetal Heimlich Maneuver that naturally expels the fluids from the lungs of the vaginally born baby.

All of these inherent safeties of pregnancy, labor and birth are signs from within ourselves as to the divine design and Creator of all things!

> *"...ON EARTH there are signs [of God's existence, visible] to all who are endowed with inner certainty, just as [there are signs thereof] within your own selves: can you not, then, see?"* [Qur'an 51:20-21]

These are just a few examples of some of the seldom seen or considered intricacies of the perfect design and inherent safeties of the reproduction process. It truly is better to follow the plan as designed and trust in our Creator, than to fumble around and interfere unnecessarily. This is not to say that medical interventions don't have their place, but when they become the norm and are done as a matter of routine protocol, we have crossed the line and actually cause many of the complications we then set out to fix. *Allah* knows what we know not.

> *"...God knows, whereas you do not know."* [Qur'an 2:216]

As you can see, if one stops to ponder the many miracles of the childbearing cycle, the inherent safety nets built into birth by our Creator become evident. Of course, any of these natural protections can be lost or maximized as a result of the mother's time and efforts to educate and prepare herself, as well as by the actions and attitudes of her prenatal (before birth), intrapartum (during birth), and postnatal (after birth) care providers. This goes hand-in-hand with the many choices the mother makes, or leaves up to others to make for her. Perhaps the most important of these decisions includes: what she eats everyday, how much she works to maintain strength and flexibility, and who will preside over her care and where her birth is planned to take place.

Taking a moment to respect the _Natural_ process is enough to bring you to your knees in submission to the greatness of _Allah_. With that submission comes the preparation needed to maximize these safety nets through good nutrition and self-care. Why would you want to mess it up with drugs and unnecessary medical interventions? _Natural_ birth is safe for the majority of women and is even more assured when she takes steps to maintain her health and prepare herself for it, _in sha' Allah_.

CHAPTER 21

Birth is Not without Risk

Despite the fundamental safety of birth, there are also unavoidable, as well as iatrogenic (doctor or attendant caused illness or injury) risks involved. Of course, underlying medical conditions, poor nutrition, and lack of physical fitness can significantly increase the risks. The key is to maximize the _Natural_ safeguards while minimizing the avoidable risks.

It's important that we trust _Allah_ and turn to HIM for help first and foremost. Unfortunately, the current birthing culture in much of the world places far too much trust in medical management and attempted control of birth. But we must accept that no own, save _Allah_, truly controls this miraculous event.

Prenatal Tests

One issue that comes to mind is the myriad of laboratory and other tests performed as a matter of routine during pregnancy. Some of these are virtually harmless, such as maternal blood draws and urine analysis, which may help identify potential problems that can support needed changes in dietary nutrition or physical activity. This might include low iron levels, sugar or protein in the urine, or the presence of a urinary tract infection.

Ultrasound

However, other tests are only seemingly harmless, as they are not proven undamaging, such as ultrasound. The issue here is that more study needs to be done before we can confirm the safety of these tests. Interestingly, the US Food and Drug Administration warns against ultrasound unless *medically necessary*.

"Although there are no known risks of ultrasound imaging and heartbeat monitors, the radiation associated with them can produce effects on the body," says Robert Phillips, Ph.D., a physicist with FDA's Center for Devices and Radiological Health (CDRH). *"When ultrasound enters the body, it heats the tissues slightly. In some cases, it can also produce small pockets of gas in body fluids or tissues."*

Phillips says, *"The long-term effects of tissue heating and of the formation of partial vacuums in a liquid by high-intensity sound waves (cavitation) are not known."*

Medical Necessity

The trouble is that the doctor may very well feel that checking on the baby with ultrasound every visit is *"medically necessary."* For example, one doctor I was following during my midwifery training was performing an ultrasound on every single pregnant mother before even looking at her chart or speaking to her.

After about the sixth woman I asked, "So, will we be doing an ultrasound on <u>every</u> woman today?"

He responded, "Yes, that way I can check on the heartbeat and see everything I need to know without ever looking at or touching the woman."

I truly didn't know how to respond to this. Seriously, I think the man is in the wrong profession! This surely cannot be considered a medically valid reason for the use of ultrasound technology!

You may want to consider this: **is there anything that can be seen via ultrasound that can be corrected if found? If not, what would you do**

with the results? Would you abort the child? What about in late pregnancy? Will "knowing" now versus later really make that much difference?

Realize, too, that there is a margin of error and "knowing" is still just "guessing." So what if the test is wrong? Even the use of ultrasound to "date the pregnancy," in order to estimate the due date, or estimate the baby's weight has a high margin of error.

Is it worth worrying about for months and subjecting yourself to the stresses and fears of that which *Allah* keeps hidden?

"...He [alone] knows what is in the wombs..." [Qur'an 31:34]

Allah truly is the best of planners and I'd suggest extreme caution when considering attempts to outsmart HIS plan, *a'uthubillah* (I seek protection in *Allah*).

I personally lived an example of this with my second child. My doctor was writing a prescription for a "Cadillac" ultrasound, as he called it. When I asked what that meant he told me that he had an ultrasound machine in his office, but since my insurance would pay for a 3-D scan we may as well go to the imaging center and get a better picture for our baby book! I have to wonder what his kickback was for referring patients for the more expensive scan, *astaghfirullah*, may *Allah* forgive me for my suspicion. But seriously, I wondered why I only "needed" this upgraded scan if my insurance was willing to pay for it?!?

To his dismay, I refused the ultrasound all together. He was totally perplexed and questioned my reasons. I replied that I wasn't convinced the test was medically necessary and that I'd rather not subject my baby to ultrasound waves that may hold some potentially unknown consequences, even if those consequences are not immediately noticeable to the naked eye. I explained that I simply don't trust the technology to be completely innocuous and have concerns that it may alter cells or genetic code that may not even be discovered until generations later, as is the case in some other seemingly safe obstetric practices of generations past (Google® thalidomide, history of pelvic x-rays during pregnancy, DES Daughters, off-label use of Cytotec for inductions, etc.).

"But what if your baby hasn't got a brain?" he asked in complete seriousness.

"Can you fix it?" I replied in question.

"No," he stated.

"Then why do I need to know now? I'm sure we'll figure that out when the time comes," I confidently replied. As a side note, this absurd statement stuck with me for the rest of my pregnancy. In fact, one of the first things I said at the moment of birth was, "Does she have a brain?" How sad that in his attempt to bully me into an unnecessary procedure, most likely for the sake of his commission, he had left me with fear and concern of something extremely rare and obscure.

Amniocentesis

What's even worse, in my opinion, is the suggestion or even pushing of tests that are known to have grave risks to the pregnancy, such as amniocentesis. This test can cause miscarriage of a potentially healthy baby. It is often offered to mothers of "advanced maternal age," as there is an increased incidence of Down's Syndrome associated with the mother's advancing age.

Doctors who suggest this will vary in terms of which patients they suggest it to. Some doctors begin offering it to mothers over 35; others wait until 40. But I have to wonder, if there is also a consideration for insurance coverage in the offering as well.

Ask yourself again, would you abort? If not is it really worth the risk to the pregnancy to find out? And, what if the test is a false positive? Is it worth the worry and stress for nothing? And what if it is truly positive? Is there any reading or preparations you can do before birth that can't quickly be done after?

Medications Increase Risk

Anytime a medication is introduced into the birth process there are increased risks and possible side effects, some of which can be life threatening. This even includes the seemingly harmless IV line, which was discussed in Chapter 3. If the birth can be accomplished drug free, why risk it? Keep in mind that generations of women before you, as well as many of your sisters today, have given birth without pain medications; with a little preparation and determination, you can most likely do it to, *in sha' Allah*!

Below is an article posted on my Saudi Life Motherhood column about your obligation to Take Responsibility for all procedures done to you and your baby. Get educated, ask questions, and read labels. Use your doctor as a resource, but not the only resource. Unless the issue at hand is an urgent matter of life and death, take responsibility for decisions made for your care. Remember, it's only you and your baby that live with the consequences, be they good or bad.

Take Responsibility

IF you read my articles on the Motherhood column you will quickly find that I advocate for personal accountability in birthing. This means taking responsibility for getting educated and preparing for birth and not just handing your body over to a doctor like you would your car to a mechanic.

It shouldn't surprise you, then, that I also advocate the same (or maybe more) accountability in parenting. This applies not only to health care you may seek for your children, but also to educational content, teachers, schools, entertainment, and general care givers.

I often speak of women in labor as vulnerable. In fact, I spend a great deal of time training fathers about her needs and prepare them to advocate and protect their wives during pregnancy and birth. How much more, then, do our children, who are not only vulnerable, but also completely innocent and dependent, need such protection?

Starting at Birth

From the moment of birth there are dozens of decisions being made on behalf of the child. These can be made by the parents or by the medical staff, who are far too often given carte blanche authority to reign over the child's treatment and care.

I really encourage parents to snap out of the daze of labor and pay attention to what's happening to their baby. Do you really want all of the routine procedures administered by your health care provider? Did you even ask, prior to the birth, what protocols are in place for your baby? Have you researched any of them to determine if you agree to them?

In this article, I'm not offering my opinions about the choices you have. I'm simply pointing out your obligation to protect your child by making informed decisions. It's important that you realize that making no decision is effectively making the decision to hand over your responsibility to someone else, who may be acting out of protocol, which may not be in sync with your desires for your child.

The list is endless, but here are some examples:

Newborn Routines

1. Pulling on the head during delivery
2. Timing of cord clamping and cutting
3. Suction of mouth, nose, stomach
4. Separation from mother/nursery observation
5. Bathing
6. Dressing
7. Formula feeding/use of pacifier
8. Prophylactic eye drops
9. Vitamin K injection
10. Vaccinations

Pediatric Medical Care

After birth, the responsibility and choices grow as the child does. You have the same issues crop up every time you take your child for medical care, whether they are ill or for a check-up. Did you interview your pediatrician and ask about their education and philosophies? Do you ask about procedures and injections before they are administered? Do you ensure that medical staff wash their hands and wear gloves before tending to your child? Do you watch them open sterile packets before use on your child? Do you read labels or research the side effects? Or do you simply hand your child over with the sentiment that doctor knows best? Your child is counting on you to ensure that whatever treatment is given is the best for him/her. Do your part to be informed before you consent to anything.

Below are some suggestions in *The Bradley Method® Student Workbook* to consider before consenting to medical care (for any medical situation, no matter who the patient is).

Informed Consent

1. What are the reasons the drug or procedure is being proposed?

2. What are the expected results?

3. Are there other options?

4. What are the possible side effects? [Be leery if the answer is "none."]

5. How will the benefits outweigh the risks?

6. What is the risk to refusing the treatment?

7. How long can we wait before doing it?

8. Can we have some time to research and discuss this?

9. What subsequent treatment or procedures will become necessary after this?

10. Get a second [or third, or fourth] opinion!

Education

But the decisions don't end with medical care. What about education? Have you ever browsed (let alone truly read) your children's curriculum? Do you know what they are learning in school?

What do you know about their teachers? Have you met the staff at the school, including teachers, administrators, and cleaning crew? Have you asked your children about the things their teachers say or how they are treated in school? If your children are young, do you know and trust the person in charge of assisting with toileting? Have you ever spent a day (or more) volunteering and observing the classroom, halls, or recess?

It is unnerving to know that Saudi law does not require criminal background checks of the people that work closely with children (required at least in schools by many other countries). Not that background checks are a complete safeguard anyway. But with the realization that many child predators seek out employment in schools or other places where children congregate (like daycares, theme parks, and family restaurants) is reason enough to blatantly trust no one!

In fact, the Canadian Centre for Child Protection warns, "...***sex offenders seek employment and volunteer opportunities within child-serving organizations as a way to access kids***....*If organizations aren't equipped with the knowledge and skills to identify risk, then the kids in their care will continue to be at risk. Criminal record checks and background checks are not enough.*"

Entertainment

What about the ways in which your children pass time? Do you know their friends? Do you know their friends' parents? Are you aware of where they hang out and what they do? What about the media they choose (television, movies, music, Internet)? How about the books they read or games they play? Do you ever stop to watch, or read, or play what they do? Do you ever say, "No," or limit their activities (especially as they mature)?

Caregivers

Possibly one of the most amazing to me is the regular use of nannies and maids in Saudi. These women are often given total reign over children for hours on end. I've actually heard people say that they don't trust their maid to cook for them (for fear she may do something nasty, or poison their food), yet they place a newborn baby in her arms and walk away without a second thought! This just makes my head spin!

158

What about the morals and behaviors of the maid? Be they general or religious, do they match yours? How can you be sure? Do you realize that your child will pick up the ways, habits, and beliefs of those who care for them? Is this maid someone you truly trust to raise your child and instill values and influence the character of your children?

A friend who works as a private tutor once told me that the wealthy preteen children she worked with confided in her that they loved their maids more than their parents. This is not surprising, considering that the maids are the ones who spent the most time with them. Do you really want someone else raising and nurturing your child?

Conclusion

This is not written to point fingers or cast judgment. Believe me, this is directed towards my own family, first and foremost! I simply want you to think about why you had children and how you want to raise them. Parenting is a huge responsibility and the obligation is one we will answer for on the Day of Judgment. As the Prophet (*sallallahu alayhi wa sallam*) taught, we are all responsible for our children and as the *Qur'an* teaches, our children are test for us.

Abdullah ibn Umar reported that he heard the Prophet Muhammad (*sallallahu alayhi wa sallam*) *saying: "Every one of you is a guardian, and responsible for what is in his custody. The ruler is a guardian of his subjects and responsible for them; a husband is a guardian of his family and is responsible for it; a lady is a guardian of her husband's house and is responsible for it, and a servant is a guardian of his master's property and is responsible for it. A man is a guardian of his father's property and is responsible for it so all of you are guardians and responsible for your wards and things under your care."* (Bukhâri 3/592)

"Your riches and your children may be but a trial: whereas Allah, with Him is the highest Reward." [Qur'an 64:15]

Guard Your Health

Keep in mind, there is no such thing as a risk free birth. Just as there is no such thing as a risk free walk in the park. Every step and every breath of life is a gift from God. It's prudent to heed the advice of the Prophet's (*sallallahu alayhi wa sallam*) when he said to prepare for the future in the *hadith* below.

> *On the authority of Abdullah bin Umar, who said: The Messenger of Allah took me by the shoulder and said: "Be in the world as though you were a stranger." Ibn Umar used to say: "At evening do not expect [to live till] morning, and at morning do not expect [to live till] evening. Take from your health for your illness and from your life for your death."* [Bukhari]

It doesn't take much consideration to recognize that the physical condition in which a mother enters labor will have a significant impact on her birth experience and recovery period afterwards. With careful attention to a well-balanced diet and simple exercises designed to prepare the pregnant woman's body to function at its best during her labor and birth, we are taking the most important steps at minimizing risks by maximizing potential. It just makes sense that the healthier and more physically and emotionally prepared the mother, the better her outcome will be, *in sha' Allah*.

As has been discussed in earlier chapters, good nutrition and physical activity cannot be underestimated. In fact, these are the two most important factors to healthy outcomes and they are also the two the mother has the most direct influence over during her pregnancy. Also noted before, there are no "redos" in the baby's growth and development. This "no redo" theory also applies to the birth experience.

Don't just ignore the approaching birth and leave your outcome to chance in the hands of mortals. By not preparing you effectively up the risks. Take care to prepare yourself and your baby while you can in order to remain healthy and low risk and be careful where you place your trust for this _Natural_ life event.

Chapter 22

Birth is Not without Pain

No matter how you arrange it, there will be some pain associated with birth. Some mothers are better at rearranging their perception of pain to that of discomfort or even positive progress, but the physical sensations are intense, nonetheless. There is even a small trend towards the extreme of seeking sexual pleasure during birth; however, I have yet to see that in person. In most cases, the total submission and complete vulnerability to the process of birth that would be needed to achieve an orgasmic birth is out of reach. I will note, however, that birthing in water seems to be a key factor in reaching that plateau, or close to it.

Medical Mercy

The medical establishment prefers you not to have pain during labor. I suppose this is quite merciful, *masha'Allah*. Besides that, a painless patient is a passive one. Not to mention that a patient strapped to monitors, IVs, and epidural drips is much more complacent and easier to deal with than one who remains active and aware of her sensations. Of course, this pain "free" birth comes at a high price. This is a price that you are paying, not your doctor.

The truth is that a medical birth does cost more money. This directly affects hospital and care provider profits and incomes. But aside from that, the even higher price is the increased risks to the health and welfare of the baby. But that's no problem for the hospital staff; they simply strap the monitor on and prepare for the possible emergency surgical birth that will serve to further increase profit and income, *astaghfirullah*.

Downsides to Medical Pain Relief

But let's back up a moment and consider these points:

1. Medicinal pain relief may not come when you feel you need it most. Most women experience a good portion of their labor before the medication is administered or takes effect. How will you cope with the pain until your drugs are administered and take affect if you're not prepared?

2. Medicinal pain relief may not work, or may not work as well as you hope. Many women still feel pain, even under the influence of pain medication. Many think that it's just an isolated incident and the medication just didn't work for them. But this issue is more common than most realize. In fact, one of my students confided that her epidural only numbed one side of her body, she still felt all of the pain and sensations on the other. Of course, there are no refunds in cases like hers.

3. Sometimes the pain medication itself comes with its own set of pains. Epidural can leave women with backaches, headaches, obsessive itching, and more for hours, days, weeks, or even years after birth. These are just the minor complications. That's not even the tip of the iceberg when you consider some of the major ones, including permanent paralysis and even death. On top of this are the extra procedures that are done to a woman under anesthesia that are often far more invasive than for a *Natural* birth because she can't feel to push properly or get into the best positions. The added delivery "help" that comes because of her inability to birth on her own are more likely to leave her hurting when the pain meds wear off. But this is the mother's problem, to deal with alone

at home, far from the care of the medical staff that sold her the "relief" to start with.

4. Many don't realize that the submission to epidural comes with an increased risk to mother and baby. Evidence of this can be seen in the required IV (just in case an emergency ensues), mother's blood pressure must be monitored more often because the meds may have dangerous effects on her heart, the baby's heart rate must be continuously monitored because the drugs reach him or her within sixty seconds and are often times culprit in fetal distress. But that's okay, right?!? After all, the doctors are ready and waiting with their knives to quickly fix the problem via cesarean. Personally, in most cases, I don't think trading the pain of labor, as prescribed by *Allah*, for a handful of increased risks, is a smart move unless there is some medical indication besides normal labor pains. Everyone has to bear their own pain, but I trust that *Allah* will not give us more than we can handle as noted in the four *ayats* (verses) listed in Chaptr 8:

"God does not burden any soul with more than he is well able to bear..." [Qur'an 2:286]

"... We do not burden any soul with more than he is well able to bear......" [Qur'an 6:152]

"...We do not burden any soul with more than he is well able to bear..." [Qur'an 7:42]

"...God does not burden any human being with more than He has given him - [and it may well be that] God will grant, after hardship, ease. [Qur'an 65:7]

5. Of course it's rare that women truly understand that the epidural also comes with a cascade of other interventions. Besides those noted in number four above, are you aware that you may be catheterized with epidural? This means a long tube is inserted in the urethra (the tube leading from the genitals to the urinary bladder) so that urine can be drained manually, as you will no longer have control of your bladder or bowel. Did you know that since you

can't feel to push your baby out, epidural may greatly increases the risk of delivery by forceps or vacuum extraction (tools used to manually pull the baby out by his head)? Of course, these tools will require extra room in the birth canal, so you can bet you'll be getting a nice-sized episiotomy (surgical cut in the vaginal tissues) to go with that! Sure, you might not feel all this, but do you really want it? What about after the pain medication is worn off? I am sure you'll feel the aftereffects! And who wants to feel horrible when it counts most, when the new baby is in your arms? Wouldn't you rather take the pain before the birth and feel victorious and virtually pain free after? You can surely rearrange the pain, but it's never truly gone.

I wrote two related articles on the Saudi Life Motherhood column. The first is "Should We Rearrange the Pain?" and the other is "12 Epidural Realities."

Should We Rearrange the Pain?

ASK any woman who has bore a child about her experience with labor and birth and two things will most likely hold true:

She will be able to tell you every little detail, even decades later.

She will not be able to tell the birth story without mentioning the PAIN!

These things will remain consistent, regardless of whether or not she opted for pain medication for her delivery. Of course, depending on the type of pain medication administered, she may or may not remember everything, but what she does remember will surely include pain.

There are basically three types of anesthesia given for childbirth pain "relief": local, regional, and general.

"Local" refers to the numbing medication given at the "local' site of the pain. For birth it is administered by a needle injected into the genital area during the pushing stage of labor. Its purpose is to numb that area so that the mother does not feel the baby passing out of her body, or to numb her for the surgical cut (given far too routinely) that widens the opening and makes it easier for the baby to pass. This anesthesia does not prevent her from feeling the pain of the contractions nor does it prevent her from effectively pushing to assist her body with the delivery.

"Regional" refers to the medication given by injection into much deeper tissues or cavities to numb a much larger "region" of the body. The widely used epidural is a "regional." It is administered by inserting a needle into the epidural cavity near the spinal cord. It prevents the woman from feeling any sensations from her waist down and she typically becomes immobile from the time it is administered until it has worn off. It's important to note that it also relaxes the uterine muscles and hinders her ability to push effectively.

"General" refers to the medication given that renders the patient completely unconscious so that medical procedures can be performed while she sleeps. It is commonly administered as a gas via a breathing mask, or intravenously through an IV. With this type of anesthetic, there is no way the woman can work with her body to push the baby out.

In the article *Drugs, Myths and Birthing* printed in The Bradley Method® [of Natural Childbirth] Student Workbook, Jay Hathaway, Executive Director of the American Academy of Husband-Coached Childbirth® raises some interesting points about the "myths" surrounding birthing and the use of pain medications. Some quotes from the article include:

- *"Birth is not without pain. Birth is never without risk."*

- *"Pain can be minimized, rearranged, changed or postponed...but I doubt it is ever truly gone."*

- *"...in labor women make noise, and he [referring to an obstetrician] was trained to make them quiet by giving them drugs to 'shut them up.'"*

- *"Has silence been mistaken for pain relief?"*

- *"...mothers [who plan ahead of time to take pain medication] did not learn any of the many natural, effective techniques for handling pain in labor because they expected the drugs to 'work' and assumed they would feel no pain. By the time they realized the drugs were not going to render their labors painless, they were helpless to do anything else."*

- *"All drugs used in childbirth are dangerous...they [can] have serious* effects...[or even] disastrous effects on the baby and the mother..."

- "...[there is very little] difference between cocaine and the drugs used for epidurals...all of them...[are] caines just like cocaine. All these drugs belong to the same chemical family."

- "How can street 'caines' be bad but, medically administered 'caines' be harmless? The chemical effects of the drugs are the same, regardless of the source or the intentions of their administrators."

- "All obstetrical pain killing drugs have been proven to reach the unborn baby, including epidurals. (Anesthesiology 29:951)...epidurals and even so-called locals 'may result in significant neonatal drug exposure.' (Am. J. Obstet. Gyne-Col. 149:403)"

- "...no drug...has ever been proven safe for the unborn baby."

- "All childbirth pain medications...do reach the unborn baby, usually within one minute."

- "An epidural...may relieve the pain before birth but it can leave the mother paralyzed and in pain for hours after the birth, and sometimes...can last for days or longer."

- "The majority of anesthetics are administered into very sensitive areas of the body with very long needles...'pain-relief' can actually be quite painful [to administer]."

- "A lot of things in life are painful, and yet, nobody uses anesthetics for them. Ever watch a baseball player crash into the...wall to catch a dumb little ball and save the game?...[He doesn't] ask for drugs..."

- "Drugs decrease performance. What have you ever done that could be more important then giving birth? Drugs mess-it-up."

I can tell you from my personal experience of giving birth naturally eight times, (without any pain medications or medical "intervention") that the pain of birth is over the minute the baby is born, *alhamdulillah*. Sure, I feel pain up until that point, but it's nothing I couldn't handle by applying the natural techniques I had learned in Bradley Method® childbirth classes about coping with pain in labor and working with my body.

I can also tell you that I've seen many mothers coming out of the delivery room after a medicated, so-called "painless" birth. Those are the mothers that are moaning and groaning, groggy and sick. They are miserable at the moment when they should be overjoyed and eager to care for their newborn baby.

My experience, and that of other natural (non-medicated) mothers I've seen, is that we feel great when it matters most, when our baby is placed in our arms for the first time. We typically are up and walking immediately following the birth. Most of us "_Natural_ moms" are ready to go home from the hospital with just a couple hours of restful bonding time in the recovery room.

"_Natural_ moms" also have far less interventions; interventions which cause bruising and injury to our bodies and require a great deal of healing after the birth. It is far less joyful to care for and bond with your new baby when his/her birth is the source of the misery and pain a mother must deal with afterwards. Most "_Natural_ moms" feel great and have nothing to "recover" from.

Sure, we can delay or rearrange the pain with drugs. But do we really want to? Do we want to move the pain from a few hours _before_ the birth to a few days or weeks _after_? Think about it...how you choose to deal with the pain of your labor and birth will not eliminate it, but will seriously affect the outcome and how well you feel during those precious early days with your new baby. _Allah_ (_SWT_) prepared the perfect plan for our labors, maybe we shouldn't interfere!

---

12 Epidural Realities

SOME women love their epidurals (medication administered straight into the epidural space near the spinal cord during labor to numb the body from the waist down so that she doesn't feel her labor or birth). But I wonder how many have considered the added risks and realities before they consent to it, or the cascade of other interventions that happen once it is administered.

Did You Know:

1. The medication used for epidural is a narcotic (in the same family as cocaine)?

2. The medication reaches your baby within sixty seconds?

3. There will be extra procedures and possible complications done to you because of the epidural?

4. Due to the increased risk of fetal distress caused by epidural, your baby's heart rate must be more closely monitored (why put your baby at added risk)?

5. Due to the increased risk of maternal blood pressure problems, your blood pressure must be more closely monitored (why put yourself at added risk)?

6. You will have no control over your bladder or bowel and may therefore be given a catheter (long tube inserted into your urethra that stays in place to keep your urine drained into a bag that will be hung under your bed)?

7. Having a catheter increases risks of bladder infection after birth?

8. The epidural will likely slow your labor and make it longer?

9. You will likely be given synthetic hormones to make your contractions harder due to the relaxing effect the epidural has on your womb muscles and these harder, drug induce contractions are more stressful on your baby?

10. If you can sit totally still during contractions so that they can administer the drug, you are probably strong enough to handle your labor without it?!?

11. Some women get no relief from epidural at all, yet it still adds all the increased risks to their baby and there will be no refunds!?!

12. If you Google "Epidural Accident" you will find over 700,000 results?

First Hand Epidural Accident Story

I want to share with you the story of someone I know personally. She lives in the United States. Like many mothers, she fears the pain of labor and likes the idea of drugs to numb her instead. In fact, she fears the pain so much that she schedules her baby's birth a couple of weeks before her due date and goes into the hospital for her epidural and then induction. In this way, she skips even the first few contractions and she is perfectly happy with that.

This worked well for her first two births. However, when she went in for the third something went wrong. Somehow, the epidural numbed her from the nose down, rather than the waist down. Suddenly she couldn't breathe; her lungs were paralyzed by the epidural-gone-wrong. This phenomenon, called pulmonary paralysis, although rare, is one of the more common epidural risks.

Thankfully, in her case, fast action was taken by her medical team. The obstetrician did a bedside cesarean delivery while the anesthesiologist worked to insert a tube down her throat and hooked her up to a breathing machine that breathed for her until the epidural wore off. This was a true emergency and the quick work of her medical team saved hers and her baby's lives.

However, since it was done in such urgency, the sterility of the procedure was not maintained and she and her baby ended up with severe infections after birth. In fact, they both almost died after the birth and were very sick and on strong antibiotics for about six months.

What's most ironic to me is the mother's response to this. She told me, "Thank God for my doctor! Can you imagine if I had considered a home birth? My baby and I would have died!"

I'm just shaking my head and thinking, "Really?!? You're grateful that your hospital induced emergency was solved by the same people who caused it in the first place?" I'm sorry, but from my perspective there's some missing logic in that one!

Get Educated

Even if you are sold on the idea of an epidural, get educated about the risks and benefits before making a final decision. Also consider at least trying to go _Natural_ and see how it goes. If you take the time to learn how to work with your body and to prepare for the birth you just might find that you don't need the epidural and all it's risks after all. Besides the education won't hurt and you might learn some valuable things for your journey to motherhood that you'd miss otherwise.

First Hand Regret

Another mother in Saudi bluntly told me, "I don't need your childbirth classes because I am going to ask for the epidural in the parking lot!"

I was fine with that, after all, it's her baby and her birth, not mine. But after the birth she was singing a different tune.

"Oh, Aisha, I wish I had taken your classes!" she lamented.

Come to find out, when she got to the hospital in strong labor she was not given her epidural right away, despite begging for it, because her insurance did not cover it. Her valiant husband rushed downstairs to pay for it, only to realize that it was Friday, _Jumu'ah_ (prayer time). For those of us in Saudi, we know what happens to the cashiers at _Jumu'ah_: THEY CLOSE!

The poor husband ran frantically around the hospital trying to find anyone to consider his plight and take his money. No one seemed to care. Finally, he resolved to returning to the cashier counter to wait, only to find himself eighth in line!

At last he paid and rushed back to his wife waving the valuable pink receipt to save the day, only to find out that the anesthesiologist was now back-logged and his wife was third on his list.

"Aisha, I was begging for my epidural for a couple of hours before I got it! I so wish I had taken your classes so that I'd have at least some clue what to do for my pain during that time. I really felt helpless and with my husband out of the room I was even more panicked!"

Considering the Realities

Now that you know some of the realities of the "magic" epidural, I hope you might think twice about it. Childbirth really isn't all that bad if you learn how to work with your body and prepare for it. Trust me, if it were so unbearable I would not have eight children, *subhan'Allah*!

AMANI Birth Classes

We now have Islamic childbirth classes that teach about birth as worship and trust in *Allah* (*SWT*). At the moment they are offered in Riyadh, but will soon be spreading all over the world as new teacher trainings are being scheduled in several locations, including Saudi Arabia, Malaysia, Indonesia, Egypt, and USA, *insha'Allah*.

If you'd be interested in classes or becoming an AMANI Birth Teacher, visit http://www.amanibirth.com for more information. The *Ummah* (*Islamic community*) needs more sisters helping sisters through education during this special time in their lives.

Natural Ways to Minimize Pain

Although birth is most likely going to hurt, keep in mind that every woman has the power to minimize her pain _Naturally_. We have already discussed many of these empowering tips:

1. Work with your body to minimize pain (maintain active upright positions while you can, relax in forward leaning positions and let your body work when labor gets strong, staying off your back and out of stirrups, etc.).

2. Ignore your labor for as long as possible (the longer you can maintain your normal activities, the shorter your labor will be).

3. Keep up your energy by resting if it's your normal sleeping time.

4. Eat early in labor while you can. When you can no longer eat, keep eating a small amount of dates and stay hydrated with water. Dates

are full of iron and are a good source of quick energy. They also provided calcium and vitamin K, both of which are necessary for proper blood clotting, thereby minimizing risks of postpartum hemorrhage, especially if eaten as a part of the regular pregnancy diet. Recall the birth of Isa/Jesus:

...*"Grieve not! Thy Sustainer has provided a rivulet [running] beneath thee;*
and shake the trunk of the palm-tree towards thee:
it will drop fresh, ripe dates upon thee.
Eat, then, and drink, and let thine eye be gladdened!..."
[Qur'an 23-26]

5. Avoid unnecessary pain by utilizing total relaxation with deep, calm abdominal breathing. Submit to *Allah* and let go. This will allow your body to do the work at hand during the hardest parts of labor while minimizing pain. Total relaxation really will cut your pain in half (or conversely, tensing up and fighting your labor will double your pain).

6. Utilize positions for the actual birth that will minimize the muscular effort needed to push your baby out. Upright positions utilize the force of gravity. Especially squatting, which not only opens the outlet of the pelvis by about 30% as compared to lying on your back, but also shortens the birth canal. If you end up in a more recumbent position (semi-sitting or simulated squat on the delivery table), be sure not to spread your legs far apart for the birth. Instead, pull your knees back by holding your legs under the knees and pulling back, keeping your elbows up and out. This will work with the anatomical design of the genitals and allow the perineum the most stretch. If you allow your legs to be spread far apart, as with stirrups, you risk tearing and will most likely be given an episiotomy anyway.

7. Be determined to give birth to your baby! Submit to the power of *Allah* and resist the temptation to submit to medical interventions unless you experience a serious complication, which is far less likely if you have taken the time to prepare and have remained healthy and low-risk with good nutrition and exercise.

Conclusion

So although birth is not without pain, we do have control over how much pain. We also have control over how we perceive the pain, which effects how much it hurts. We also have control over when that pain is most intense. I'd venture to advise that taking the pain before the birth, as prescribed by our Creator, is a better bet than after pain medications have worn off and we are left to heal from unnecessary medical interventions.

Chapter 23

Dangers of Interventions

I am the first to acknowledge the skill and efforts of our medical establishment at rescuing mothers and babies in trouble. I'm very grateful for medical interventions when they are truly needed. In most cases, true need for interventions is related to underlying medical conditions or lack of preparation on the part of the mother. But for the vast majority of healthy, young women, interventions cause more harm than good. Especially when they interfere with the _Natural_ process and lead to a domino effect of more and more invasive measures. Many of these unnecessary interventions have been mentioned in previous chapters.

Medical "Truths" Change

Medical science is constantly making new discoveries in the arena of pregnancy and birth. The truth is that what was thought to be safe yesterday, may be known to be harmful today. Consider some of the obstetrical history noted in prior chapters and the changes that have taken place over the years as we discover the harmful effects of some of the seemingly safe test, medications, or procedures that were once routine for most pregnant or laboring women.

When you take into account that there is always room for human error, I have to ask, **"Why risk it?"** I truly trust that *Allah* didn't make any mistakes when HE designed our reproductive process. Unfortunately, in our desperate attempt to control that which is out of our control, coupled with our own ignorance of the delicate balance at play in <u>Natural</u> birth we end up interfering and often times messing things up.

Hospital Protocol and Routine

The first thing to realize is that much of what is done to a woman in labor is a matter of routine and protocol. Some of it, actually I'd venture to say much of it, is totally unnecessary. In fact, routines come and go, some falling by the wayside. But then I am shocked to find some that have become passé to be revived in sparse pockets of the birthing community here and there.

Some examples of this are routine enemas and shaving of the pubic hair upon admittance for birth. These were common procedures decades ago that are so out-of-date that they are rarely ever heard of now. Yet I was shocked to find at least one hospital in Saudi still clinging to these totally unneeded procedures that serve only to humiliate the dignity of the mother.

The important thing for you to recognize is that you don't have to submit to everything they "offer" and can refuse "care." But you must pick and choose your battles, because if you become too adversarial and "combative" then your birth team will find it difficult to want to support you in your birth plan at all. It's a balancing act between what they are used to doing, what really needs to be done, and what you are willing to put up with.

It's a good idea to discuss routine protocols, procedures, and prepping standards with your doctor ahead of time. This way you can come to an agreement about what you do and do not agree to and ensure there is a note in your file (and your hand) stating that the specific routines you are refusing are excused. This is also a good gauge to determine if the doctor of choice will support your birth plan. If it's a struggle to discuss minor routine protocols, you might want to shop around for someone more in tune with your birthing ideas.

Vaginal Exams

One of the first things they will want to do upon your arrival at the hospital is a vaginal exam to assess your labor. No woman submits to vaginal exams without some embarrassment and discomfort. You need to understand what is the purpose of the exams and that you can refuse them if you want. After all, the baby will be born, *insha'Allah*, exam or not. Of course the doctor will insist and even be stressed without the information from the exam. I am not telling you to accept or refuse, but consider what they are worth and what they risk and then make your own informed decisions about them.

First of all, expect some pain with the exam, especially if the doctor insists on doing them during contractions. They do this to assess what the baby's head is doing in relation to the contractions. Whether or not this information is "necessary" is a matter of opinion. Of course it may also be the hinge of deciding whether or not to "allow" you to labor naturally or to step in with drugs, procedures, and surgeries to deliver the baby. Here is where it's important to have done your shopping around before labor to find a doctor you trust so that you do not find yourself second-guessing everything they do or say. A relationship of mistrust between patient and doctor can be deadly.

Secondly, you should know that there are four basic pieces of information being gathered during vaginal exams. It's important to realize that this is limited and subjective information. The four measurable factors include the following:

1.   Effacement of the cervix (the thinning of the connection between the womb and the vaginal canal).

2.   Dilation of the cervix (the opening of the connection between the womb and the vaginal canal).

3.   Determination of the part of the baby that is presenting first as well as the angle it is presenting. This means checking if the baby is coming head first or buttocks first, as well as the relationship of the back of the baby's head as compared to the mother's pelvis. The most normal is the "LOA" or left-occiput-anterior position, which means that the back of the baby's head is facing the front-left of the mother's pelvis. This information can be helpful in understanding why a mother might be having a more difficult or

prolonged labor, as posterior positions (when the back of baby's head faces mother's spine) are harder, can be more painful, and typically take more time.

4. The station or level of the baby as it passes through to the mother's pelvis. This information is deemed important for doctors to estimate if the baby is making progress through the hipbones. To assess this the examiner will imagine a line across the prominent spines of the lower pelvis. If the presenting part (hopefully the head) is in line with spines it is said to be at zero station. If it is above the spines it is at a negative station (negative three means approximately three centimeters above the spines); if it is below the spines it is at a positive station (positive three means approximately three centimeters below the spines).

It is important to realize that every examiner has a potentially different assessment based on his/her experience and subjective evaluation of the factors being measured. In fact, a doctor I was shadowing during my midwifery training confided that it took him about 50 to 75 vaginal exams before he felt confident in what he was doing, and that even now he's only about 80% accurate.

Yet this information could be used as the basis for interventions, including surgical delivery. You should also know that each exam increases the risk of infection, especially if the bag of waters has ruptured. This is true even though sterile examination gloves are usually used. In fact, some care providers do not do exams at all due to the infection risks, discomforts, and their opinion that the information gained is not essential.

If assessing progress were a necessary factor in birth, you'd have to wonder how generations of babies were born before medical interference existed. Not only that, but there are other, noninvasive ways to assess progress in labor. Not to mention that these four things are not the only progress being made, as discussed in Chapter 19.

Frankly, an attendant who pays close attention to the behaviors of the woman, her modesty as it declines, the shape of the abdomen as the baby moves down, etc. will have a good sense for what is happening. There are also external physical signs of cervical dilation that can be observed, such as a darkening line that rises up the backside of the mother's buttocks as the cervix opens, but I doubt an hospital attendant would know about this or attempt to use it to assess dilation.

The important thing here is that your choices about consenting or refusing vaginal exams be respected. Your decision about whether or not to accept vaginal exams may change during labor as your desire to know what's happening internally can override your concerns about the discomfort or risks of infection. Additionally, vaginal exams can give very essential information when labor is long and hard, as sometimes the baby may be entering the pelvis in slanted (asynclitic) manner and at times the attendant can help adjust this malpostion manually. However, in the majority of cases, with or without a vaginal exam, your baby will be born on its own, *insha'Allah*.

My biggest advice is to tune into your body and trust *Allah*. If you sense things are going well, you can probably trust that. However, if you have a sense that something isn't right, follow that and seek guidance from your care provider. Remember that the providers you have chosen are there to support your birth and help you with the knowledge they have gained through study and experience. Use them as the resource they are, as this is an appropriate reason for hiring them in the first place.

Mother's Position

Requiring a mother to assume a certain position in labor and birth is almost always detrimental. She should tune in to her body and assume the positions that feel right to her. Of course we've already discussed the importance of mobility and also how placing a mother on her back and in stirrups causes harm to her and the baby (decreased blood flow, altered blood pressure, increases risk of fetal distress leading to cesarean, fights gravity, increases incidence of tears or need for episiotomy from spreading the legs too far apart, closes the pelvis by up to 30% as compared to squatting, etc.). Yet this ludicrous position is often forced on women for the convenience of the attendant.

Realizing that positions that are best for the doctor are not always best for the mother and baby should be enough to motivate women to advocate for themselves on this important issue. Stay mobile and off your back and do what's best for you. After all, the birth should be all about the mother and baby and the care provider should never be the focus of the event.

Fetal Monitoring

Fetal monitors use ultrasound waves to record the baby's heartbeat simultaneously with a recording of the intensity of the mother's contractions. I've already discussed my concerns with ultrasound technology in Chapter 21. I'm therefore not too keen on subjecting my baby to hours of ultrasound exposure during labor.

Not only that, but the device itself is uncomfortable, as the external fetal monitor is comprised of two hard boxes that are strapped to the mother's abdomen with Velcro belts. This may be okay for an epidural mother, but for a _Natural_ birth mother they add to the discomfort of the contractions. On top of that, they virtually render the mother immobile, as she is strapped in bed to the machine, often on her back, which you already know by now is the worst possible position. Not to mention how vitally important freedom of movement is in labor.

Of course, there is also an internal fetal monitor. This device has a small copper screw at one end that is inserted into the womb via the birth canal and literally used to pierce the baby's skin and is then screwed into the head. I'm sure it's probably not much more invasive than a pin prick, but I don't like this idea at all! Not to mention that by piercing the skin it opens a pathway for infection. To top that, the bag of waters must be broken first, if not already done. Artificial rupture of membranes is another intervention I'd rather not submit to.

Another thing to consider is that it is a machine and machines can fail. There have been cases of faulty readings that lead to surgical deliveries of perfectly healthy babies. Also realize that the reason they were invented was to reduce the incidences of cerebral palsy brought on by lack of oxygen during the labor and birth. In retrospect, the rates of cerebral palsy were not reduced at all. In fact, all we got was increased medical interventions in births, including more cesarean deliveries, and no better outcomes than when we monitor with low-tech devices and the human eye and ear.

Moreover, I'd venture to say that we get far better care from human observation than we get from mechanical monitoring.

One case I was witness to involved a mother carrying twins. I'm not sure why she came for observation, but she was sent to the nurse who was running electronic fetal monitors for outpatient women. She was having a hard time picking up the heartbeat of one of the twins and came to a senior nurse midwife for assistance. I happened to be following that midwife during my clinical studies as a midwife trainee. As I stood back watching, I witnessed these two nurses fiddling with the straps on the mother's abdomen and the dials on the machine. Understandably, a twin pregnancy poses more difficulty using the machine, as you must ensure you are picking up each individual baby's heartbeat. I could see one of the babies was registering a heartbeat within the normal range and the second, although present, was much below the expected range for a fetal heartbeat. I didn't think much of it at the time until I was told the next day that the mother was taken for emergency cesarean many hours later and lost one of the babies. Looking back, I felt saddened that no one picked up a manual Fetoscope to listen to that baby in distress. We could see it on the monitor but the nurses were so busy trying to "fix" the machine that they didn't accept or recognize that it truly was a baby in distress. I have no idea if the time wasted would have made a difference in saving this baby and I am not blaming the staff. Obviously we must accept the decree of *Allah*. However, it really made me realize that when we put our total dependence on a machine we lose touch with the woman and her baby. There really is no replacement for human senses and direct observation.

Besides this, the monitor is only as good as the person monitoring the monitor. If we strap women up to machines and thereby accommodate more patients per human nurse, we reduce the amount of direct assessments made with human observation, intuition and care. There are even cases that have gone to court where the monitor has picked up on real complications but no one was checking the monitor, so there were grave outcomes despite the information regarding the baby's distress being recorded continuously. Had there been no monitor, there most likely would have been more frequent staff observations, as the low-tech monitoring requires human presence.

Just remember the benefits and risk equation when making decisions about accepting or rejecting any aspect of care. How do you feel about the procedure? Have you done research about it? Don't just trust my advice, there are plenty of online resources to consider. Also ask your doctor's opinions and reasons. Be sure to get facts and don't be afraid to ask for written studies to back up his/her practice.

Intravenous Infusion

IVs administered solely as a matter of routine are really not needed in the case of a healthy, normal labor and birth. Chapter three highlights many of the pitfalls to having an IV line running, especially with glucose. But one thing that is not mentioned is the effect it often has on the baby. When the mother's blood is circulating high levels of glucose, the baby also must deal with the artificially raised blood sugar. As a result, the tiny pancreas works overtime to keep producing insulin in order to cope with the elevated blood sugar.

But what happens when the baby is born and the umbilical cord is cut? At this time the source of the increased sugar is terminated. The baby now has too much insulin circulating in its blood and becomes dangerously hypoglycemic, at which point he/she is rushed off to the NICU (neonatal intensive care unit) and bottle-fed glucose water to help stabilize the blood sugar. This removes all chance for immediate breastfeeding, and all of the benefits that accompany it, interrupts the precious first hours of bonding, and can also lead to nipple confusion and difficulty initiating breastfeeding afterwards.

Not to mention the fact that having an open line to the mother's vein makes it far too easy for medications to be given without informed consent, especially in countries without informed consent laws. Keep in mind that you have a right to know what is being administered to you, why, what the risks are, what the expected benefits are, and most of all you have the right to refuse anything that is not occurring as a matter of urgency with regards to life or death.

As noted in Chapter 3, complete avoidance of an IV may not be the top priority in your birth plan. In fact, if you sense that you are in for a lot of self advocating you should pick and choose your battles and save your energy for bigger things. So long as you remain well hydrated and are low risk, you may want to consider consenting to just having an IV catheter inserted without running a drip to it. This will allow the medical staff to administer medications quickly in the event of an emergency, while still giving you control over gaining information about what's being given so that you can give true informed consent or refusal before anything is administered. The thing to remember is not to be too quick to surrender your rights or your health during what should be a *Natural*, normal life event!

Inductions, Augmentations, and Elective Cesareans

Classic examples of often-unnecessary interventions are induction or augmentation (speeding) of labor as well as scheduled cesareans near the end of pregnancy. Some doctors are of the belief that terminating the pregnancy before *Natural* labor starts is a good idea. In fact, it allows them to schedule your birth within their busy schedule and ensures that the assisting staff on hand are those most competent and easy for him/her to work with. It is also better business, as cesarean surgery pays more than attending a *Natural* birth and takes far less time. It also lends a sense of control over that which only *Allah (SWT)* truly has control.

Their mind set is often that you've reached a point in your pregnancy where the baby's body systems are mostly developed and there is little visible risk to the baby, who will most likely thrive outside the womb now, *in sha' Allah*. They also fear a pregnancy that goes "post date" may be a potential problem. While this is sometimes the case, it is often a matter of wrong pregnancy dating to begin with. My preference is to wait on *Allah's* timing; however, I'd seriously consider *Natural* measures to prompt labor before consenting to medicinal ones.

Something for the mother to consider when faced with suggestions or orders for induction or augmentation are the fact that the contractions brought on by medical means during an induction or augmentation of labor are not the same as *Natural* contractions. They are much stronger and do not adjust based on your body's signals or tolerance. Due to the stress that they often cause to mother and baby, there will be much closer monitoring of both, along with a readiness to "rescue" you with cesarean in case the induction "fails." Most mothers also do not realize that an induction is not an instant process. If you go in for an induction, prepare to room in for a while, as sometimes it can take up to three days, especially if the cervix isn't "ripe" to begin with.

The truth is that forcing labor to start, especially with medicinal agents, increases risks to mother and baby. It also ups the chances of emergency cesarean, which escalates the overall risks again. Not only this, but it interferes with the final days of growth that cannot be "redone" outside the womb. In fact, the final days of pregnancy are most important for brain development. That's not to say that your child will be "less than normal" if born a few days early, but it's safe to say that we are stunting the intrauterine growth and limiting the maximum potential that was slated for this child. There are also plenty of cases where an elective induction or cesarean has resulted in unintentional prematurity due to miscalculated size and dates.

Speaking of due dates, it's important to realize that they are just an educated guess, not an exact science. For more on this topic I've included an article I wrote on Saudi Live, Your Due Date and Inductions.

Your Due Date and Inductions

FROM the first moment a woman realizes she's pregnant she wonders, "When am I due?" In fact, this may be the most anticipated piece of information that her care provider will tell her during her first prenatal visit. Additionally, it is probably the most frequently asked question she will hear in the coming months. As her pregnancy progresses, it may also become the most anticipated date of her life!

Fortunately, there is scientific research to provide an *estimated due date*. This is typically done by calculating approximately forty weeks from the woman's last menstrual cycle. Additionally, measurements taken during an ultrasound scan are used to estimate the gestational age of the baby. There are also other, less scientific methods, for guessing the due date. These can include calculations based on the mother's first notice of fetal movement, among others.

History of Due Dates

Interestingly, the most commonly used method is based on the research of a German doctor in the 1800s. His findings are what the forty-week gestational period is based on. But it's important to note that this assumes a twenty-eight day menstrual cycle. It becomes increasingly inaccurate if your cycles do not fit into his assumption of a *normal* twenty-eight day cycle. In fact, a Harvard public health study indicated an average gestation of forty-one weeks plus one day. This study suggests that the date given by your care provider is likely to be eight days early!

Ultrasound Dating

Ultrasounds give us the ability to measure the baby's growth. The ultrasound software then *estimates* the due date by comparing these measurements against a *normal* range for size. It's important to note, however, that every baby grows at a different pace. In fact, it is logical to consider that shorter parents might just have smaller babies than taller ones. Because of this, ultrasound dating is considered less accurate the further along the pregnancy is. In fact, early ultrasounds have a margin of error of approximately plus or minus six days and late term ultrasounds have a margin of plus or minus two weeks!

Probability of Due Date Delivery

Most care providers will acknowledge that the due date is only an educated guess and consider two weeks on either side of the date to be within *normal* range. Realistically, your chance of spontaneous birth occurring on your due date is only about 4%; whereas the probability of delivering within thirteen days either side of your due date is roughly 70%. That still leaves an over 25% chance that you will deliver more than two weeks before or after your due date.

Importance of Due Dates

It's important that expectant couples take note of the word *"estimated"* when considering their due date. A due date really is nothing more than an educated <u>guess</u> as to <u>approximately</u> when your baby <u>might</u> be born. Notice all of those ambiguous words?

This is especially important information for couples who are encouraged to consider a scheduled induction of labor. Because I am not a doctor, I can never advise you with regards to your particular medical situation. Therefore, I would never tell you what you should do. But I do want parents to be informed of the very *normal* range of gestation so as not to be rushed into a decision that carries increased risks to the health and safety of both mother and child.

Scheduled Induction

It is of major concern to me when I speak to expectant mothers, time and time again, who are being encouraged or advised to schedule an induction. Typically the suggestion for induction starts at about thirty-eight weeks gestation (two weeks before the *estimated* due date). The suggestion for induction will usually get stronger and more demanding as her *estimated* due date approaches. If she reaches, or passes, her *estimated* due date, the suggestion for an induction may become more of an order or a threat, than a suggestion.

I personally must question the agenda when the medical provider starts discussing medical management of the birth date, especially prior to the *estimated* due date. If the pregnancy is healthy and uncomplicated, my concern turns to the doctor's trust in the <u>*Natural*</u> process.

Unfortunately, if the doctor in question does not trust birth, he or she will be inclined to medically manage as much of the process as possible. In my humble opinion, this is a sign that he/she has a fear of birth to the point that they feel a need to dominate and control every aspect of the event.

Trust Birth

As an advocate for _Natural_ birth, I would not want to put my trust and body in the hands of such a provider. Personally, I trust _Allah's_ design of our bodies and accept the fact that birth is unpredictable and much of it uncontrollable. I also recognize the many inherent safeguards that our Creator has built into the pregnancy and birth process. Having said that, I also understand the value of childbirth education. Learning about these safeguards allows us to prepare for birth in order to work with our bodies to maximize them.

Respect for Doctors

In all fairness to doctors, I must express my respect for their training in pregnancy and labor abnormality. They are the experts and our safety net when complications do arise.

Additionally, true postmaturity is an illness and means more than simply past _estimated_ due date. In fact, it is a real risk for babies as the placenta ages and is not able to adequately nourish the baby. However, only seven percent of babies go beyond forty-two week gestation. Even of those that do, true postmaturity is extremely rare.

As for the perception of their need to manage or control the birth process we should consider three factors:

1. Medical training teaches about complications and interventions to reduce risks and save lives. Often times, doctors prefer induction because they can't guarantee that something bad might not happen if they wait.

2. Since they are trained to intervene, many doctors never actually observe or participate in completely _Natural_, non-medical births. Because of this, they may find it hard to trust the _Natural_ process.

3. Most women lack understanding of the _Natural_ birth process. Therefore they are unaware of the many safeguards _Allah_ (SWT) has provided for us in birth. Without this knowledge they do not prepare their bodies physically, nutritionally, mentally, and emotionally to work with these safeguards and ensure each one is available at peak performance. As a result, many cases

seen by doctors are of high risk, unfit mothers who are not at optimal preparation for _Natural_ birthing.

Induction Risks

It's utterly important that expectant parents realize that there are medical risks to induction. So long as the mother is healthy and doing well and there are no medical signs of fetal illness, I believe patiently waiting is far safer than medical induction, _Allahu A'lam_.

Induction of labor literally means a medical _attempt_ at forcing the early termination of the pregnancy. I use the word "_attempt_" because there are no guarantees of success and the risk of Cesarean section delivery is therefore greatly increased (as much as fifty to two-hundred-fifty percent). Below is only a small list of the myriad of risks to labor induction on both mother and baby:

1. Abnormally strong, frequent contractions

2. More painful contractions for mother

3. Fetal distress for baby (may be reason for Cesarean)

4. Increased risk of infection to both mother and baby

5. Umbilical cord preceding baby during birth, as labor may be forced before baby engages into the pelvis (can cause fetal death)

6. Uterine rupture caused by over stimulation of the muscles (especially if the mother has previously had a Cesarean delivery)

7. Possibility of allergic reactions to medications used for mother and baby

8. Domino effect of increasingly invasive medical procedures, including Cesarean

Informed Consent

Obviously, there are cases where delivery is safer than continuing the pregnancy, for mother or baby or both. However, it's important that parents have full disclosure of the reasons for suggesting the induction as well as the real risks and benefits so that they can assess what's best for them.

Ultimately, it is the parent's right and obligation to weigh the risks. They are the ones responsible and must come to their own decisions regarding their care and acceptance of medical interventions. After all it's the parents, not the doctor, who live with the consequences of the risks of induction verses the risks of continuing the pregnancy until spontaneous labor begins.

Preparation for Due Date

As we wait for our due dates there are many preparations to consider. Personally, I feel the mother's physical, mental, and emotional preparation for labor, birth, and motherhood is of top priority. Additionally, I am an advocate for fathers at birth; but only if he is willing to lovingly support his wife and takes the time to get educated.

Childbirth education and lots of reading about birth, labor options, and breastfeeding top my list of things to do. However, there are also the more tangible, and probably more fun preparations to consider as well. These may include:

• Preparing the baby's room

• Stocking the baby's wardrobe

• Selecting baby's furniture

• Purchasing baby accessories

• Installing the car seat

• Choosing a name, etc.

Conclusion

One thing is for sure, assuming we live through the pregnancy, birth will come, one way or another, *in sha' Allah*. One other certainty is that there is usually plenty of time between the discovery of the pregnancy and the *estimated* due date to get educated and make the necessary preparations for labor, birth, and parenthood, *alhamdulillah*.

God knows what any female bears [in her womb], and by how much the wombs may fall short [in gestation], and by how much they may increase [the average period]: for with Him everything is [created] in accordance with its scope and purpose. [Qur'an 13:8]

I also find it a fitting reminder for *Ramadan*. We need to work hard to be prepared for our *estimated* due date. Yet the actual date a baby will be born is known to no one, except *Allah (SWT)*. How similar is this to our need to work hard to be prepared for our ultimate date with *Allah (SWT)*? After all, this date is also known to no one, except HIM. The difference is that we may not live to see our baby's birth date, but we shall surely be present when the trumpets are blown and each of us will surely see Judgment Day!

Even though it may sound good to get it over with, especially for a mother who is weary towards the end of her pregnancy, she should seriously consider the risks of inductions and cesareans before making the decision to consent. The first priority should be welfare of the baby. If the baby is tolerating the pregnancy well and the mother is fine, then just wait it out. *Allah* (*SWT*) knows best and it's prudent to trust HIS timing in all things.

Another thing to recognize is that even spontaneous labor can be rushed along with the same drugs used for inductions. These drugs are often administered when your progress in labor is not as fast as the doctor would like, or as hospital protocols dictate. Sadly, these drugs are sometimes given to almost all women as a matter of routine. This is called augmenting or speeding labor. Remember that these drugs have a domino effect that often lead to higher and more invasive measures, including cesarean section. In fact, they often lead to the two reasons often cited for emergency cesarean. The first is "Fetal Distress," which can be caused by induction or pain relieving medications (often taken as a result of the increased pain from the induction drugs) as well as the resulting immobility of the mother. The second is "Failure to Progress," which is often referred to as "FTP." In the world of *Natural* birth advocates, "FTP" often means "Failure to be Patient!"

Natural Induction Measures

For those mothers who feel that they are being pressured or bullied into an induction, I'd suggest a second or third opinion. You may also consider some of the *Natural* measures you can try when you feel pressured to finish the pregnancy before spontaneous labor begins. Most won't do much if the body isn't already "ripe" and near ready, but then again, often times the medicinal inductions "fail" if the body isn't already "ripe" and near ready too!

One of the least invasive *Natural* induction techniques is sexual intercourse. The nice thing about this is that it will have no effect unless the woman is ready for labor anyway. One factor is mild contractions that come with female orgasm due to the release of oxytocin hormones. Similarly, stimulating the nipples produces oxytocin hormones, which cause contractions. If the woman is about ready to start labor, these sexually induced contractions may just do the trick at kick starting the process. Another factor has to do with the hormone present in male semen, which helps to soften the mother's cervix if it is "ripe" and near ready for labor. The hormones in semen serve this *Natural* purpose as the mother's receptors to the hormone peak just before labor. This is a reason why medicinal induction on an "unripe" cervix, which often begins by applying a synthetic version of this hormone to the cervix vaginally, is often "unsuccessful" and likely to lead to a cesarean delivery.

Acupressure points are also valuable in prompting *Natural* labor. But unlike intercourse, care should be taken not to undergo these measures unless you are truly past your due date. The last thing you want is premature use of acupressure, which could result in a baby born much too early. The points to consider are noted below:

1. Press your thumb against the roof of the mouth, like an infant sucking her thumb.

2. Find spleen 6 on the lower leg, shown by the red dot on the drawing below. It is a noticeably soft and sometimes tender spot a couple of inches above the ankle bone on the big toe side of the leg, this area can be pressed and massaged for several minutes at a time

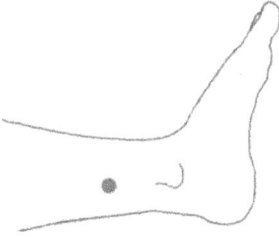

3. Find bladder 60 on the lower leg, shown by the red dot on the drawing below. It is on the pinky toe side of the leg, located between the protruding anklebone and the Achilles tendon. You can press into this area, which should be like a valley. This is especially helpful for a baby who is high in the pelvis and hasn't "engaged" yet. Often times the doctor will refer to it as a "floating" baby.

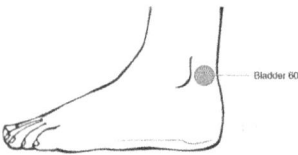

Bladder 60

4. Find bladder 66, on the outside edge of the pinky toe, shown by the black dot on the drawing below. This area can be pressed with your finger or thumbnail and is also good for bringing a baby down, particularly if the mother is stressed or has fear and anxiety about the birth.

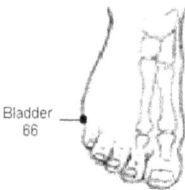

Bladder 66

5. Use the palm of your hand to rub quickly, back and forth, across the instep of the foot, as shown in the photo below. This movement should produce a heat, like rubbing kindling for a fire. This is

particularly helpful for mothers who have retained water or are overweight.

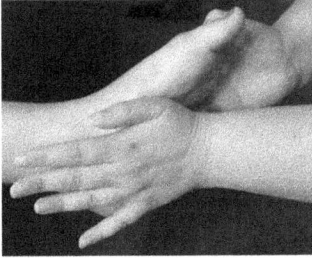

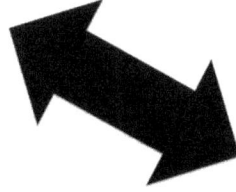

Reflecting on the alternatives, _Natural_ birth that begins and ends spontaneously is by far the healthiest route for both mother and child. When we begin to alter the birth process by medical intervention, we also begin to alter the outcome. Interventions bring a new set of risks to mother and baby as well as affecting the bonding period after birth. Many interventions also introduce a need for healing and recovery that would not have occurred otherwise. In some cases, the benefits of intervention outweigh the risks, however, in the majority of healthy, normal pregnancies, the _Natural_ route produces the healthiest outcome.

Breaking the Waters

The baby is surrounded by a sac of amniotic fluid, often called the bag of waters, during pregnancy. This bag of waters typically breaks sometime during labor, although it may break prior to the onset of labor. Few people realize that in rare instances it doesn't break at all and the baby is born still enclosed in the intact amniotic sac. This rare occurrence is called being born in the "caul" and was thought to be a sign of nobility in some ancient cultures.

However, it's rare that a baby born in the hospital could ever be born in the caul since doctors are keen to intervene and break the bag of waters during the labor. This is mostly an unnecessary intervention and it can cause the baby to drop down into the pelvis in a bad position.

Doctors like to break the water as it can help bring the baby's head into stronger contact with the cervix and may increase the rate of cervical dilation. It also facilitates the doctor's assessment of the baby's presentation, as it's easier to feel the baby directly during a vaginal exam than with a bag of water between the examiner's fingers and the baby. Additionally, it allows the doctor to assess the clarity of the fluid. If it contains fecal matter of the baby, it may be a sign of distress (although often is completely normal and not a sign of stress at all).

I personally prefer allowing *Allah's* timing to pass and therefore letting the waters break (or not) when it happens *Naturally*. As with accepting any type of intervention, you must make your own decision based on the information you have at the time. It's not wise to be so stuck on any particular point that the health and safety of mother or baby are at risk. The advice here is to be flexible, but not blind. Be educated ahead of time, ask questions at the moment, and make the best-informed decisions based on your particular case and after weighing the risks and benefits. As always, healthy mother and baby come before everything else.

Cord Clamping

Somewhere in distant history obstetrics adopted a protocol of routine and immediate clamping and cutting of the umbilical cord after birth. There has been a lot of controversy in recent years about the potential harms this practice causes to the baby. We have many studies that report the benefits of delaying this action, at least until the cord stops pulsing, or better yet, waiting until the placenta is born. There is even a growing trend today for parents to choose not to cut the cord at all. They simply carry the baby and placenta together until it falls off naturally. This practice is called "Lotus Birth." Interestingly, allowing the *Natural* process to take place without clamping and cutting the cord reduces the time of the umbilical cord falling off and healing from one to two weeks, down to about just three days.

> *"The suggested neonatal benefits associated with this increased placental transfusion include higher haemoglobin levels (Prendiville 1989), additional iron stores and less anaemia later in infancy (Chaparro 2006; WHO 1998b), higher red blood cell flow to vital organs, better*

cardiopulmonary adaptation, and increased duration of early breastfeeding (Mercer 2001; Mercer 2006). There is growing evidence that delaying cord clamping confers improved iron status in infants up to six months post birth (Chaparro 2006; Mercer 2006; van Rheenen 2004)."

In fact, World Health Organization and the International Federation of Gynecology and Obstetrics (FIGO) have dropped immediate cord clamping from their guidelines. Yet most doctors still do it. Those that do are clearly not practicing evidenced-based care in this regards and it leaves me to wonder about all other aspects of their care as well. I suppose that the old ways have become habit and the benefits of delaying the cord clamping just haven't struck them as important enough to change.

Personally, I feel that the practice of immediate cord clamping is an injurious insult to the mother and baby. Some of the less measured benefits include:

1.   Keeping mother-baby intact as a unit ensures bonding and encourages breastfeeding.

2.   Much gentler transition to lung breathing for the baby as he/she continues to receive oxygenation from the mother during the first tenuous breaths.

3.   Gentler and better psychological transition for the baby, who is ensured to be with mother, as compared to being born and whisked away, handled by rubber gloves, placed on a hard surface under bright lights, being poked and prodded, all during a time when the greatest instinct is to find the breast.

4.   If the baby's breathing is compromised and there is a need for resuscitation, the intact cord Increases oxygenation from placental supply, which can be massaged and "milked" even after it has been expelled from the mother's body.

Also consider that the placenta and umbilical cord contain about one third of the baby's blood. By clamping the cord prematurely the baby is effectively robbed of this stem cell rich blood that belongs in his/her circulatory system. No wonder it takes six months for the child to recover the lost hemoglobin!

The picture below illustrates the transformation of the umbilical cord over a period of about 10-15 minutes after birth. Note how thick the still-pulsating cord is in frame one, compared to the same segment of cord as it becomes limp and thin by frame six.

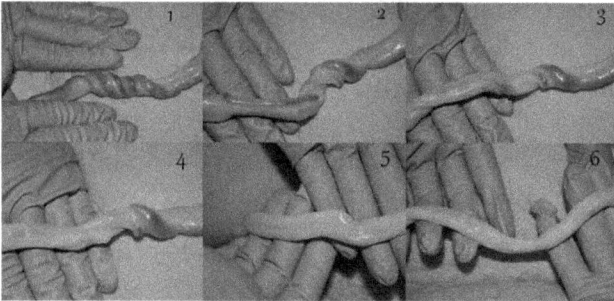

Borrowed from Nurturing Hearts Birth Services
(http://www.nurturingheartsbirthservices.com/blog/?p=1542)

On a personal note, when I had my first baby, my husband was offered the opportunity to cut the umbilical cord, as is customary in America. When he did so he couldn't help but comment, "Wow! That's really tough, like a garden hose!" I didn't think much about it at the time but I have remembered this all these years. Obviously, it had been immediately clamped and was still thick and pulsating, as in the first frame of the photos above.

Ironically, when I had my eighth baby at home with my second husband, I instructed him on where and how to clamp and cut the cord. We didn't do this until forty-five minutes after birth and by then the baby was breathing just fine and had nursed several times, *masha'Allah*. He was not aware of the comment of my first husband so many years before, yet he couldn't help but comment as he cut the cord, "Wow! That's smooth, like silk or butter!" *Subhan'Allah!* What a difference it made to delay cutting the cord until the baby was finished with it, as he hadn't clamped or cut it until it was more like the last frame of the photos above!

I suddenly felt my heart heavy as I realized what I'd allowed to be done to my first seven children. Thankfully, they are all healthy and fine, but I can't help lament that it could have been a better start for them, had I just known and advocated for my baby's right to go straight to breast and delay the clamping of the cord until it is finished pumping.

Coincidentally, the eighth baby was extremely even tempered and relaxed in her infancy. Frankly, all my children were good babies, but she was exceptional, *masha'Allah*. She was really the most relaxed, content, and simply the least demanding baby that I have ever encountered. I truly believe that it has a lot to do with the gentle and uninterrupted transition into this world that she experienced, *subhan'Allah*.

Assessing the Harms

It is difficult to evaluate the extent of individual harms caused by medical interventions since we can never really measure for any one family the alternative outcomes once interference begins. However, it shouldn't take much consideration to realize that anything successfully accomplished without the influence of drugs and knives will have a healthier, more Natural outcome.

Just keep in mind that medical interventions may have their place and time, but also that each and every intervention introduces new risks. There are never any guarantees that interventions will deliver the desired outcome or that they won't make things worse. The biggest peace and comfort comes in knowing that absolutely nothing passes without *Allah's* leave and that HE promises that with every hardship comes ease.

> *"Say: "Nothing will happen to us except what Allah has decreed for us: He is our protector": and on Allah let the Believers put their trust."* [Qur'an 9:51]

> *"...God does not burden any human being with more than He has given him - God will grant, after hardship, ease.* [Qur'an 65:7]

CHAPTER 24

Points to Minimize Interventions

As noted in Chapter 3, women are their own worst enemies in terms of achieving a _Natural_ birth by placing their trust in medical management and pharmaceuticals before trusting _Allah_. Submitting to pain medications messes up the _Natural_ process and really does not bring better outcomes. Medical staff often make matters worse by pushing pain drugs to keep the labor wards quiet, after all, this makes patients far easier to manage, regardless of the increased risks to mothers and babies. Remember this is your pain and your rewards and expiation of sin, not theirs, and giving you drugs to silence you or keep you complacent is not in your best interest.

Abu Hurayrah (Radiallahu Anhu) reported that the Prophet (Sallallaahu 'alayhi wa sallam) said: " Whenever a Muslim is afflicted by harm from sickness or other matters, Allah will drop his sins because of that, like a tree drops its leaves." [Bukhari, Muslim]

Abu Sa'eed al-Khudree (Radiallahu Anhu) reported that the Prophet (Sallallaahu 'alayhi wa sallam) said: "A Muslim is not afflicted by hardship, sickness, sadness, worry, harm, or *depression - even if pricked by a thorn, but Allah expiates his sins because of that."* [Bukhari, Muslim]

Remember too that lack of patience is often at the heart of many medical procedures. Have confidence and trust in *Allah's* timing and accept the term of labor HE has prescribed for you. This is better than the drugs and domino effect of interventions prescribed by doctors, not to mention the increased healing time and pain that comes with the interventions offered.

Putting your trust in our Creator's design of your body and of birth in general is the biggest step towards avoiding medical interference during what should be a _Natural_ life event. Getting educated and working to prepare for your birth are the first physical steps towards minimizing medical interventions. Good birth consumerism and selection of a supportive birth attendant and birth location also top the list. Maintaining self-confidence and determination and ensuring that your birth companion(s) share the same confidence in Allah's design (and in you) will go a long way towards achieving a completely _Natural_, drug-free birth, *insha'Allah*.

Keep a confident and positive attitude. Work with your body to minimize pain in a _Natural_ way and accept the blessing of expiation for what's left over. Considering each moment of discomfort as a necessary step in the journey to motherhood will keep your mind free of the torment that breeds increased tension and pain. Submission to *Allah's* decree always makes hardships easier.

Also keep focus on the baby's birth experience. Barring serious complications, which are rare in a well-nourished, healthy mother, the _Natural_ process is almost always better and far gentler. Many medical interventions come with the risk of fetal distress, which is a direct ticket to cesarean delivery and trauma for both mother and baby.

Remember the Creator's design for after birth as well. The benefits of immediate breastfeeding are numerous. Don't worry about getting "dirty" from holding your baby fresh from the womb; you can shower later! Put the baby straight to breast, even while the cord is still intact. This is a _Natural_ way to control your after birth bleeding and expel the placenta, as well as providing the best start in life for your baby.

As discussed in Chapter 11, the first substance to come from the breasts is called colostrum. It is often referred to as "liquid gold." The small amount of colostrum produced is a perfect match for the tiny size of the newborn's stomach (about the size of a pea). It is full of important antibodies to protect the baby in his new environment. It is also a _Natural_ laxative that helps to clear out his intestines of the first sticky bowel movements, called meconium. It provides all the nutrients the baby needs and the mother should never supplement with formula, water, or anything else while waiting for the milk to come in. Immediate nursing also reassures the baby and provides a bonding avenue of comfort as he transitions to his new surroundings.

The ten most important steps to minimizing interventions include:

1. Education and knowledge

2. Physical preparation

3. Mental and emotional preparation

4. Good choice of care provider and birth place

5. Determination to birth _Naturally_

6. Confident, loving support person(s)

7. Well thought out birth plan

8. Advocate to resist the first intervention, as it may lead to the next

9. Ask questions and speak up for your right to informed consent or refusal

10. Make _dua_ and trust _Allah_

If your birth experience does not play out as you had hoped, it's important to remember that a healthy mother and baby trump everything else. Maybe it could have been better, but what's done is done and we know that _Allah_ is the best of Planners.

CHAPTER 25

What to Expect in <u>AMANI Birth</u> Training-Part Four

The *Natural* Series focuses on trusting *Allah's* design for birth and minimizing medical interference. Having an understanding of why labor is an important part of the birth process gives new respect and honor for our Creator's plan for this *Natural* life event. Exploring the ways that drugs and medical interventions screw it up help mothers and their partners to become committed to doing what it takes to birth in trust of *Allah!*

Together they will learn to work with the mother's body to reduce pain and employ *Natural* pain management techniques. They will also discover respect for the medical process when complications do arise. But understanding that complications are rare in a normally healthy and well-nourished mother will help to maintain the determination needed to accomplish a truly empowering and *Natural* birth for the best start in life, *insha'Allah.*

The *Natural* series is compiled of four modules:

Module 1   The Purpose of Labor

In this module we will explore the many reasons for labor and its role in the journey to parenthood. Understanding that there's more to labor than can be measured by a vaginal exam is a sign within ourselves of the greatness of our Lord. We will also discuss the tendency of the medical profession to be impatient with laboring women and explore some of the benefits to surrendering to the time prescribed by *Allah (SWT)* for labor.

Module 2   Working with Your Body

In this module we reflect on how the female body works in labor and begin to recognize that labor is a physical and emotional cooperation between mother and baby. This allows mothers to purposefully choose calm and relaxing movements and actions that will help the *Natural* process, to submit to the Creator by submitting to the labor, and to be cognizant of how their behavior will help or hinder the process.

Module 3   Complications

In this module we will explore common complications and how to deal with some of them in a *Natural* manner, as well as recognize the need for flexibility and appreciation for medical assistance when it is needed. We will discuss things to consider if a cesarean does become necessary, as well as recovery tips afterwards. Trust in *Allah* also extends to trusting that nothing happens without HIS leave and that with every hardship comes ease.

Module 4   Minimizing Medical Interference

In this module we will discuss how the various pieces we've learned to-date come together to minimize your need for and likelihood to submit to medical interference. By understanding what's normal in labor and working with your body you will be well equipped to manage your labor *Naturally*, thereby reducing need for interventions, *insha'Allah*. You will also begin to consider what things are most important to include in your birth plan.

PART FIVE – INSTINCTIVE

The *Instinctive* Series focuses on trusting *Allah's* perfect design of our bodies to carry, birth, and feed our babies. We will discover the role of hormones in labor and how our emotions affect their flow. Along with this we will explore the influence our birth environment has on the process of labor.

Unfortunately, when birth became institutionalized, we transferred our trust to the medical profession and muted the innate birthing voice. Additionally, we have sent signals to women for decades that their bodies are defective and they need medical assistance to perform some of the most natural of human events.

It's time to reevaluate where we place our trust and learn to listen, once again, to the signals that come from within. When we become aware of our innate abilities to birth, we can begin to tune out negative messages and distractions in order to tune into the primitive instincts that guide us through labor. When we understand the importance of tuning into our bodies and turning to *Allah* we find that all of the intuitive instructions we need are already present for labor, birth, breastfeeding, and beyond.

CHAPTER 26

Hawaa and Maryam (Eve and Mary)

It's clear that Hawaa (Eve), the first mother, and Maryam (Mary), mother of Isa (Jesus) both had natural births. In fact, we know, without doubt that both of these important women in our history birthed without interference or medicinal "help." Their births were assisted only by the help of *Allah* and would be classified by today's standards as "unassisted childbirths." As noted in Chapter 3, we also can deduct that the women of the Prophet Mohammed's (*Sallallaahu 'alayhi wa sallam*) time were also birthing without medicinal interference, as obstetric medicine has only been with us for the past century or so.

There is an important lesson to learn from the experiences of our sisters and mothers past, as they all illustrate the fact that women and babies were created for, and have the instincts to birth. Each one of us has what we need, deep inside, to bring our children into this world, *insha'Allah*.

Moreover, I believe that the design of birth is perfect and goes smoothly for the majority of women, so long as they don't allow the influences of our modern world to interfere. This does not mean a woman should or must birth alone under a date tree, as our Mother, Maryam (Mary), did. What it does mean is that she should guard her health with good nutrition and proper exercise in order to remain healthy and low risk during her pregnancy and provide the best start in life for her new baby.

More importantly, it means that she must work hard to educate herself on the normal functions of her body during this miraculous time in her life in order to make informed decisions with regards to the myriad of well meaning, yet sometimes obstructive, medical interventions and interference that will either be offered or pushed upon her.

As women, we must never forget to take responsibility for our pregnancy and our babies. Our health and the ease of our birth experience lies, in part, in our efforts to prepare, and more on our trust in *Allah*. Remember the responsibility and the power of making informed decisions about all events related to your care at this time. You are the only one who can control which interventions are performed by your consent or refusal, and you are the one who will live with the consequences.

Remember your instincts that are deep within and tune-in to allow them to guide you every step of the way. Seeking "expert" advice may be prudent, especially if you sense something is wrong, but blindly following is not. Weigh all the evidence to the best of your ability and make the best choices based on the knowledge you have at the time. Don't be afraid to seek second opinions and consider the risks and benefits of everything. Also remember that no one can guarantee a particular outcome and nothing will pass without *Allah's* leave.

CHAPTER 27

Emotions, Environment, and Hormones

Hormones are natural chemicals released by the body, which cause physical changes. Some hormones react to, as well as cause, extreme pleasure or fear. There are specific hormones that must flow freely in order to achieve a natural childbirth. There are other hormones that act directly against the act of birthing. If the flow of the conducive hormones are interrupted or hindered for any reason, or the adverse hormones are flowing instead, birth will likely be hindered or difficult, if not impossible. In such cases our medical providers use pharmaceutical copies of our hormones in an attempt to get the body back on track. If these fail, they are prepared to completely take over the birth by surgical means.

Emotions are strong feelings, which can affect the flow of hormones in the body. As most of us know, pregnancy itself creates a heightened emotional state wherein we are much more sensitive to our environment. The hormones conducive to birth are most responsive to a calm, serene emotional state full of love and trust. Feeling emotionally secure is important, as we must be able to let down our guard and allow ourselves to be vulnerable for our birthing hormones to flow.

Our environment has a strong influence on our emotions, thereby affecting our flow of hormones. In fact, our environment can truly make or break our emotional state and hence, affect our flow of hormones. If we feel safe and secure in our birth environment, we are more likely to be calm and relaxed, which allow us to be vulnerable enough for our birthing hormones to flow.

Oxytocin and Adrenaline

There is a delicate balance of hormones at work during the birth process. In fact, the hormones that are conducive to birth are the same hormones at play during the woman's sexual climax. The main hormone involved is oxytocin, which is often referred to as the "Love Hormone." This is a hormone of vulnerability and surrender that can only effectively flow when the woman feels loved, safe, protected, and trusts the people around her. It is considered a "shy" hormone and a sense of privacy is often needed for a woman to let down her guard enough for it to flow.

Unfortunately, the antonym to oxytocin, adrenaline, is often provoked in the modern birth setting. This hormone is often referred to as the "Fight or Flight Hormone." When a woman is anxious, uncomfortable, scared, nervous, hurt, upset, angry, or even overly excited the adrenaline hormone kicks in and renders her labor more painful and ineffective. This hormone is designed to protect the laboring women from vulnerability during threatening situations. It increases the pulse, dilates the eyes, and closes off the sphincters (circular muscles that control the exits to the bowels, bladder, and birth canal). This allows the woman to fight or flee danger while in labor. Sadly, it leaves the woman's body at odds with itself when she continues to remain in the threatening situation that evoked the adrenaline rush in the first place.

Role of Emotions

We cannot control our hormones, but our emotions greatly affect the release and flow of hormones. When you put into perspective the environment needed for the flow of oxytocin, consider the total surrender of oneself to sexual orgasm. It would probably be pretty difficult to experience a sexual climax with an audience of professionals, bright lights, beeping machines, and clinical measurements of progress throughout the process. With this in mind, it becomes clear that the modern birthing atmosphere can become a hindrance to the flow of hormones most conducive to a natural birth.

For this reason, most women labor best in their own environment, left alone (or with those they trust) to experience the occasion as the intimate event that it is. For many women this translates to homebirth, with or without professional observation and back up. For others it means laboring at home for as long as possible before heading for the hospital. For some it means learning to tune out the hospital environment and focus inward during labor.

Emotional Flashback

It's also important to realize that emotional upset in our daily lives or our past may come up during the most vulnerable moments of our birth. These unresolved emotions could bring about a disruption in our birthing hormones. This might include marital issues, struggles with our own mothers, maternal history of abuse or sexual trauma, etc. It's important to recognize potential emotional roadblocks and work during the pregnancy to resolve them before birth.

Pharmaceutical Hormones

Unfortunately, some women, especially those ill prepared for their birth experience or with deep emotional baggage, it may be impossible to find the emotional peace that is conducive to the flow of our birthing hormones. Whether the cause is environmental or otherwise, medical staff are trained to step in to take control by injecting or infusing synthetic oxytocin hormones, or by surgical delivery of the baby. In fact, hormonal drugs are given as a matter of routine protocol in some medical practices, even when there is no indication for such intervention besides speeding labor and clearing delivery beds as quickly as possible.

The synthetic pharmaceutical drugs that are available to replace our natural oxytocin hormones are called Pitocin or Syntocinon. These intravenous drips or injections bring on contractions in a very unnatural way. By using them we increase the likelihood that the women will also submit to epidural, which is a narcotic drug that comes with its own list of risks and complications. What's worse, is when women volunteer for an interruption in their natural hormone flow by requesting or submitting to epidural for an otherwise naturally flowing labor.

Dr. Sarah Buckley says, in her book, _Gentle Birth, Gentle Mothering_, *"...a laboring woman's production of oxytocin is drastically reduced by the use of epidural pain relief—this is why epidurals prolong labor. And even when an epidural has worn off, the woman's oxytocin peak, which causes the powerful final contractions that are designed to birth her baby quickly and easily, will still be significantly lessened, and she is more likely to have her baby pulled out with forceps as a result. The drug Pitocin (Syntocinon), which has been called the most abused drug in obstetrics, is also implicated. A synthetic form of the hormone oxytocin, it is used for induction and for augmentation (or acceleration) of labor. The majority of women giving birth in the United States [and Saudi Arabia] receive large doses of this drug...When a laboring woman has Pitocin administered intravenously for many hours, her body's oxytocin receptors will lose their sensitivity and ability to respond to this hormone. We know that women in this situation are vulnerable to hemorrhage after birth, and even more Pitocin becomes necessary to counter that risk."*

Environmental Influence

The delicate balance between hormones, emotions, and environment cannot be underestimated. When we disturb the intimacy of birth with a medicinal backdrop and medical protocols, procedures, and unnecessary routines we obstruct the overall flow of hormones and the progress of labor is subsequently impeded. Unfortunately, we rarely consider that it is the very environment that offers medicinal "fixes" to our bodies' seeming defectiveness that actually causes the defects to occur in the first place.

Upon further analysis, we come to the conclusion that anyone who attends a birth with the intention of observing or helping, or even worse: controlling the event, can actually make things harder for the mother by interfering with her natural flow of hormones.

Michel Odent, French physician and supporter of natural, undisturbed childbirth describes how the modern childbirth environment interrupts the natural flow of birth on his website, WombEcology.com:

> *"...the fetus ejection reflex is inhibited by any interference with the state of privacy. It does not occur if there is a birth attendant who behaves like a "coach", or an observer, or a helper, or a guide, or a "support person". It can be inhibited by vaginal exams, by an eye-to-eye contact, or by the imposition of a change of environment. It does not occur if the intellect of the laboring woman is stimulated by a rational language ("Now you are at complete dilation; you must push"). It does not occur if the room is not warm enough or if there are bright lights."*

Clearly in his description, even the presence of a well-meaning husband, doula, nurse, supportive midwife or obstetrician can derail the natural progress of birth. This does not mean that these roles do not have their place or that the woman shouldn't want them present. What it does mean is that we really have to consider our place at the birth and ensure that our presence conveys protection, support, and love for the woman, without being a force that takes over her birth with commands and instructions. There truly is a fine line between supporting and interfering.

Of course, the place of birth will play a huge part in determining each person's role at the birth. If the woman is birthing in her own bedroom, then the husband, midwife, and doula can take more of a passive and loving role and give her space and time to labor undisturbed. However, if she is in a hospital, the people closest to her will probably need to be more involved in helping her to tune out the domineering environment and provide her a sense of protection from her surroundings. Either way, she will likely benefit from the presence of those she trusts and may appreciate loving touch that conveys relaxation along with calm confidence in her natural ability to birth her baby.

CHAPTER 28

Follow Your Instincts, Trust Allah

Fortunately, we are all designed with the _Instinctive_ blueprint for giving birth and feeding our babies. It's sad that somewhere along the line we have allowed dominant procedures and medical birthing cultures to take over our natural _Instincts_. Along with this transition has come a distrust in the female body, and hence, dare I say, distrust in the Creator of all things, _audthobillah_.

Struggle with _Instincts_

Dr. Sarah Buckley, in her book, _Gentle Birth, Gentle Mothering_, discusses the struggle that takes place between a woman's _Instincts_ to birth and the myriad of instructions and orders that dominate her in the medical birthing model. She says, **"The decision to prioritize external advice above their _Instincts_ has had dire consequences for some of these women, and I conclude that, just as we have been naturally selected for our physical ability to birth, we—and all our foremothers—have been selected for our accurate _Instincts_ and intuition in birth."** She goes on to say, **"...We disempower ourselves—when we put more faith in information from the** *outside (tests, scans, others' opinions) than our own internal knowing of our bodies and our babies..."*

Just consider the animal kingdom and the multitude of women who have birthed before you. Generations of species would not carry on if pregnancy, labor, and birth were not *instinctually* safe.

Medical Safety

Many people argue about women and babies historically dying during childbirth. But how much of that had to do with lack of nutrition or sanitary conditions? How much was due to infections after the births, which are now treated with antibiotics, or congenital anomalies that can now be corrected with surgery? These medical advancements save lives, but they have little, if anything to do with the birth itself.

Maybe more importantly though, is a realization that birth is not without risk and women still die in childbirth today. Some even die because of what is done to them in hospitals. Of course, that rarely makes headlines, unless there is gross malpractice involved. When accepted routines and procedures bring about a cascade of events that result in a death that is somehow swept under the rug and considered acceptable. Fortunately, the female body is very adaptable, even to interference, and the chances of dying in childbirth are not that great for a typical healthy woman.

I am not adverse to modern medicine and acknowledge that it definitely has its place in pregnancy and birth. In fact, medical care and observation during the pregnancy plays a valuable role in screening for and treating pathologies that can occur. Prenatal care has improved the safety of many facets of childbearing. This includes:

1. Discovery of risk that is associated with a mother with an rH blood factor incompatibility with her the baby, which can lead to miscarriage and pregnancy loss if not identified and treated.

2. Discovery that urinary tract infections can lead to preterm labor and therefore stressing the importance of diagnosis and treatment of these infections promptly.

3. Sophisticated surgical deliveries that have the potential to save

mothers and babies who have true disproportion of head to pelvis, or for delivery of delicate babies with congenital anomalies who might not otherwise survive the normal birth process.

But with each of the medical discoveries, comes risk from the procedures. Even some preventative measures carry risks. Some procedures will even cause more harm than good to some mothers and babies, and in some cases the future offspring of the babies. In fact, as mentioned in Chapter 21, many obstetric procedures proved to be quit harmful to masses of babies, but those harms were unknown until they had been applied to generations of children over the course of many years. This translates to using our most vulnerable as "human-guinea-pigs."

Always remember that there is not a single drug or procedure that can be guaranteed "safe" for your baby. It is our prayer that each mother begins her pregnancy in good health and that she educates herself to make choices that will extend her good health and provide good health for her baby throughout the pregnancy, labor, birth and beyond. But never underestimate the delicate balance within the body of the pregnant woman and her unborn child. We simply cannot tamper with the intricacies of the mother-baby unit without creating an upset in some way.

Making Noise

One thing I always point out in childbirth classes is that women often make noise during labor and birth. Women may find themselves moaning and groaning or calling out. This is a very normal part of the process and we should feel uninhibited to do so. In some cases, vocalizing will unlock the strength deep within her during the most vulnerable moments of her birth.

This does not mean that she has an excuse to lose control and call out with angry or ugly words. Remember to be thankful to *Allah* and gain *hassanat* for your discomforts. In fact, labor and birth are a time for surrendering and calling out to *Allah* for his mercy. Remember to keep words of worship on your lips, such as, "*Bismillah, Alhamdulillah, ya Rabbi, ya Kareem,*" etc.

It's important that we not allow anyone to mute our births with drugs. Remember this is your birth and your pain. Everyone involved with birth should recognize that one way of dealing with discomfort is by being verbal.

Making noise is not an indication for drug-induced silence. Possibly the best support a husband can provide is loving "permission" to the mother to make noise, and the worst hindrance he can be is to panic and look to the medical establishment to fix her pain.

Trust *Allah*

Turn to *Allah* and follow your <u>Instincts</u>. Outside "evidence" is not always the best indicator of well-being or normalcy and outside "interference" does not always provide the best results. Do your own research, which includes soliciting your care provider's advice, listen to your body and your baby, and make *istakharah* to seek *Allah's* for guidance in all things.

I appreciate the advice of Dr. Sarah Buckley when she says, *"...birth is as safe as life gets and there is nothing, whether total <u>Instinct</u> or total reliance upon technology, that can guarantee a perfect outcome...for every mother and baby. Tragedy and grief are also major facets of birth, as we know intuitively."* In fact, I'd venture to say that it is the intuitiveness that life and death hold hands that leave us vulnerable and in fear for the beginning of each new human being.

Allah provides us the inner voice of <u>Instinct</u> and it is most always right. Learn to listen to that voice and to trust *Allah*. Doubts that come from external sources should always be questioned, no matter where they come from. Sometimes trusting our <u>Instincts</u> means turning to professionals for support, but at other times it means staying the natural course, despite expert advice.

CHAPTER 29

Breastfeeding and Baby Care

It is an honor and a trust from *Allah* to be blessed with the birth of a child. But caring for a new life is quite a responsibility, *masha'Allah*. There are tons of words of wisdom from those who have walked the path of new motherhood before you. But just like in pregnancy, labor, and birth, there is no greater source of wisdom than that which comes from *Allah (SWT)* Himself.

In mothering it is just as important to tune-in to yourself and your baby as it was during pregnancy and birth. Always realize that *Allah* has given the newborn the *Instincts* it needs to survive and the mother the *Instincts* she needs to provide. There is an amazing balance of dependency and provision that continually takes place between the mother and child, *subhanAllah*. At no other time is the promise of provision from *Allah* more apparent than in the proof of milk, free flowing from the mother's breasts to nourish her infant, *Allahu Akhbar*.

> *Narrated 'Abdullah: Allah's Apostle, the truthful and truly-inspired, said, "Each one of you collected in the womb of his mother for forty days, and then turns into a clot for an equal period (of forty days) and turns into a piece of flesh for a similar period (of forty days) and*

*then Allah sends an angel and orders him to write four things, i.e., **his provision**, his age, and whether he will be of the wretched or the blessed (in the Hereafter). Then the soul is breathed into him. And by Allah, a person among you (or a man) may do deeds of the people of the Fire till there is only a cubit or an arm-breadth distance between him and the Fire, but then that writing (which Allah has ordered the angel to write) precedes, and he does the deeds of the people of Paradise and enters it; and a man may do the deeds of the people of Paradise till there is only a cubit or two between him and Paradise, and then that writing precedes and he does the deeds of the people of the Fire and enters it." [Sahih Bukhari]*

Importance of a Good Start

Your birth experience has a tremendous influence on the ease or difficulties you may experience in establishing a breastfeeding relationship with your baby. Below is an article from the Saudi Life Motherhood column about how Natural Birth Increases Breastfeeding Success.

Natural Birth Increases Breastfeeding Success

ALLAH designed the female body perfectly to carry, birth, and feed babies. This miracle has been a trusted fact since the creation of humankind. It wasn't until the last century that there were other options besides natural, non-medicated birth followed by breastfeeding.

With these new options women have begun to doubt their bodies and the natural process. The introduction of medical interventions in labor and birth have produced side effects that take an irreversible toll on woman and babies. Following closely behind has come bottle feeding and man-made infant formulas.

Women have always known that with childbirth comes pain. But when we look at the modern culture of birth we find a society of women who fear the unknown pain of labor so much that they seek medical help to avoid it.

There are a precious few who still trust the perfect design of their body and choose a completely natural, non-medicated birth. These "natural moms" are also most likely to choose the natural method of breastfeeding their baby as opposed to bottle-feeding.

Fortunately, childbirth education is beginning to become available in the Kingdom, albeit sparse. Women who learn about the physiology of their bodies and the process of pregnancy, labor, birth, and lactation (and how to best prepare for it) find that they are capable of birthing their babies without pain medications and medical interventions and subsequently of feeding their babies without bottles or formula.

Unfortunately, the majority are still in the dark, blinded by the false hope for something better than nature. What they fail to realize is that the medical interventions and pain medications used for labor and birth only offer to rearrange or change the pain of childbirth, not to eliminate it. What's worse is that these modern interventions and drugs come with a myriad of unnecessary risks for both the mother and baby. Many also fail to realize the importance of breastfeeding their newborn baby, mistakenly believing that formula is just as good as breast milk.

Below are some of the things women should consider when making choices about their labors and births.

- Birth is an athletic event, which takes training and preparation. **"Birthing a baby is equivalent to swimming a mile [1.6 km],"** according to Obstetrician, Dr. Robert A. Bradley, in the video "_Bradley on Birthing_." I seriously doubt any woman could survive the swim without months of training first.

- Neither a medical nor a natural birth are painless. It's best to learn to cope with it.

- By the time pain medication is administered the woman has already spent a considerable amount of time laboring (which she probably didn't prepare for).

- Pain medications may not take away all the pain or may not work at all!

- The administration of the drug usually involves needles in sensitive areas of the body and is a cause of pain in itself.

- There are additional medical interventions that come from not being able to move or feel or push effectively (due to pain medication) which cause greater injury to the body and will be felt after the birth (and often times hurt worse than the birth itself).

- Natural birth mothers, who prepare their bodies for birth, learn to work with their labor, and employ simple techniques for minimizing pain, usually feel great after birth.

- Medicated mothers often feel nauseas, sick, and have a great deal of pain from medical interventions and feel miserable after birth.

- A mother who feels great is more capable of caring for her baby and thus more likely to breastfeed her baby right away.

The fact that "natural mothers" usually feel great after the birth, while medicated mothers do not, is of extreme significance. Do we really want to move the pain from a few hours BEFORE birth to a few hours/days/weeks AFTER birth? Think about that for a moment. You are not going to eliminate pain, but simply move it around. Wouldn't you rather feel great when it counts? When you have your newborn baby in your arms?

Mothers should also know that all medications that are used during the labor and birth of her baby do reach the baby within an estimated sixty seconds of administration. She should also know that NO medication, not even the medications used during childbirth, have been proven safe for the unborn child.

Additionally, she should realize that these medications affect her and the baby in ways that outlast the birth. Even a medicated mother who has full intention of breastfeeding may find it extremely difficult to get started due to some of the short-term effects of these medications:

- Interferes with Mother and Baby's Alertness
- Effects Mother's Ability to Care for Baby
- Causes Nausea and Other Discomforts
- Requires Prolonged Recovery Time for Mother and Baby
- Mother and Baby's Bonding Time May be Compromised or Delayed
- Interferes with Baby's Sucking Reflex Making Nursing Difficult

- Interferes with Mother's Milk Supply

There are also a myriad of medical risks associated with using these medications. Rather than making a list I'd like to ask expectant mothers, "Can you be absolutely positive that you or your baby won't have an adverse reaction to the man-made drug you are considering for your short-term comfort? Would you put your baby in harms way for a couple hours of pain relief for yourself? If you can learn how to minimize the pain and birth completely naturally, would you try?" Simply put, **"Why risk it?"**

Sadly, most expectant mothers in the Kingdom don't have the opportunity to take classes. Subsequently, they don't know what to do to prepare for their upcoming labor and birth. They are unaware of the physiology of pregnancy and birth and they are unclear about proper diet, simple exercises to prepare their body for the event, or natural techniques for coping with the pain.

These women often find themselves in a panic and unable to bear the discomforts and pains of birthing their baby naturally. They unknowingly fight their labor and make the pain worse! These women often times come into the hospital in a panic and searching for medicinal relief. In the end they feel they have "suffered through" the event and are often too sick and in pain to be able to care for themselves, let alone cuddle and nurse their new baby. The hospital staff is then left to take over and keep the baby in the nursery, feeding them with bottles of formula.

In today's medically managed birth culture it is rare for medical professionals to witness a completely natural birth. The panicked patients who seek rescue from their birth have become the norm and the calm joyous natural birth of our great-grandmothers has become abnormal.

It is a sad state of affairs when abnormality becomes normality and normality seems impossible. But it doesn't have to be this way! There is hope. As more and more women find their way to quality childbirth education there will be more and more doctors witnessing the benefits of a calm, confident, non-medicated woman, an empowered woman who confidently labors in peace.

As these women leave the delivery room touting the joys of a truly natural birth, others will listen. They will not tell of births without pain, but they have understood the process, had techniques to cope, and worked effectively with their bodies. They were in control of minimizing their pain and were able to trust the natural plan for their bodies.

They will tell of their pain being over the moment their babies were born. They will tell how they insisted on birthing completely naturally, without intravenous drips, without pain medication, even without episiotomy.

They will have advocated for their baby and insisted that the doctor delay clamping their babies' umbilical cords and that they be allowed their right to nurse their babies on the delivery table, before the placenta is even expelled. They will have acted in confidence, knowing that immediate breastfeeding is not only possible, but beneficial to both her and her baby.

These women knew that they were not in need of synthetic hormones to expel the placenta and prevent maternal hemorrhage. They learned that breastfeeding their babies produces the same hormones, naturally, that these synthetic injections provide. They knew that their breast milk is full of important antibodies that their babies need to have the healthiest start in life. They were keenly aware of the importance of bonding and nursing in the first moments of life.

What sets these "natural moms" apart is that they take the time to get educated and prepare for their births. They are determined to have the healthiest, most natural, joyous births possible. They are dedicated to their babies and insist on brining them into the world undrugged, alert, healthy, and ready to breastfeed. They are confident in themselves and understand that early breastfeeding is the best assurance to successful breastfeeding.

They are the women who will set the trend for a change in our birthing culture that will bring us back to what's worked, naturally, for thousands of years. As more women become aware of the benefits of totally natural childbirth, they will become a driving force that will create a demand for quality childbirth education. Change is on the horizon and a new era of naturally born, exclusively-breastfed babies is dawning.

Most Mothers Can Breastfeed

This chapter is not intended to be a comprehensive resource for breast-feeding or the problems that some mothers incur. However, it is important to note that the majority of women can breastfeed their babies, if given the time, patience, and encouraging support they need. Supplementing with infant formula is the first mistake mother's make when it comes to establishing a breastfeeding relationship with their baby. Sometimes it is the well-intentioned nursing staff at the hospital or the woman's own relatives who feed the first bottle in order to let the mother rest. This perceived "mercy" for the mother is actually a severe detriment in her breastfeeding success. That one bottle can leave the baby with nipple confusion and ineffective sucking at the mother's breast that does not properly stimulate her milk production.

Included here is an article from my Saudi Life Motherhood column, The "Just One Bottle" Myth.

The "Just One Bottle" Myth

AS a mother-to-mother breastfeeding counselor I often get calls or emails from nervous new mothers who worry that their milk supply isn't enough or has dried up. It's understandable to have such concerns, especially with the myriad of pressures from friends, relatives, doctors, and media to supplement with bottle-feeds.

Generally speaking, these worries are not justified. In fact, most mothers produce more milk than their baby needs and the more she nurses, the more milk her body will make.

"False Alarms"

Mothers get alarmed and attribute several myths to their worry about supply:

- Baby may change feeding frequency or habit

It is expected that baby's feeding patterns will change over time. In fact, it's very common for babies to increase feeding frequencies just before a growth spurt.

- Mother's breasts feeling less full than before

As mother's body adjusts to the sucking stimulus, she will find that her breasts do not feel full between feedings, since the milk is not "let down" until the baby suckles.

- Inability to get much milk while pumping

A lack of expressed milk may just mean that mother is not able to effectively replicate "let down" using pumps or hand expression. It's also important to understand that the mother must achieve a very relaxed state in order to release hormones in her brain that trigger her milk to "let down" (whether nursing or pumping). Often times, she just cannot reach that deep level of relaxation while pumping, as she naturally does when actually nursing her infant.

- Baby having fussy periods

Fussy periods can be caused by many factors, including nipple confusion or lazy nursing after experiencing the easy flow of artificial teats. Onset of illness or teething can also be normal culprits to baby's change in behavior.

Trust Your Body

For many women it's difficult to just trust our bodies to provide for our babies. Since we can't measure how much our babies are drinking we are vulnerable to doubts, worry, and outside influences.

However, the best determinations are the baby's output (wet/soiled diapers) and weight gain. Newborns will typically need to be changed six times per day with three or more of those being soiled changes. As babies mature, it is normal to have less bowel movements than before (usually after six weeks of age).

As for weight gain, it is important to note that babies lose up to 10% of the birth weight. If they have gained back to their weight at birth by two weeks, they are doing well! From this point until about three months they should gain 140 to 170 grams (5-6 ounces) per week.

Unfortunately, many doctors do not receive adequate training or study in lactation. Additionally, it's much easier to calm a worried mother by offering the "easy" and measurable alternative of bottle feeding during a ten or fifteen minute office consultation than spending the time it may take to counsel and reassure a breastfeeding mother who may have a hard time believing what she cannot see (amount of milk being consumed).

Expect Insatiable Nursing

Growth spurts can also be a cause for concern, as baby will suddenly seem to be hungry "all the time." Typically they occur between 2-3 weeks, at six weeks, and again at three months. Sadly, many women make the mistake of *"just one bottle"* during these times as they feel their baby's insatiable hunger is a sign of starvation rather than a natural increase in stimulation to prepare extra milk for the coming spurt.

> *"...mothers may nurse their children for two whole years, if they wish to complete the period of nursing..."* [Qur'an 2:233]

It's no coincidence that the majority of women who do not complete the full two-year nursing term tend to quit after just 2-3 weeks, or at six weeks, or at three months. I really cannot stress enough that the baby needs NOTHING but mama's breast milk for the first six months of his/her life. As I said in the article, *Relearning the Natural Way of Infant Feeding*,

> *"Nothing" really does mean NOTHING: no formula supplements, no baby cereal or foods, no juice, no teas, not even water!*

"Just One Bottle"

The biggest concern I have as a lactation counselor is the *"just one bottle"* myth. Many mothers are encouraged to get some extra rest or to leave baby with a relative and allow *"just one bottle"* of formula. *"Just one bottle"* can interrupt the establishment of milk supply and put a mother on a downward spiral towards more and more supplementing and less and less nursing.

Read what the World Health Organization and others have to say about supplements:

1. "**The administration by bottle** and teat of water, herbal teas, glucose solutions or worse still, milk-based formulas, **not only is unnecessary on nutritional grounds, but reduces the infant's sucking capacity and therefore the mother's lactation stimulus.** Furthermore, such practices increase the risk of introducing infection and in the case of milk-based formulas, of sensitizing an infant to cow's milk proteins!" --Joint WHO/UNICEF Statement, 2006

2. "Babies who are fed by bottle are likely to suck the breast in the same way. "Nipple sucking", in contrast to "breastfeeding", means the baby does not open her mouth and attach to the breast in a way that effectively removes milk and causes breastfeeding hormones to be released. Mothers of babies who have been given bottles often get sore nipples and make less milk because their babies are nursing ineffectively. Pacifiers can cause the same problem. **Even one bottle can interfere with breastfeeding. The risk of interrupting breastfeeding increases with the number of bottles given.**" --Responsibilities of Health Workers under the International Code of Marketing of Breast milk Substitutes and WHO Resolutions, 2009, ICDC

3. "**Breast milk is the only necessary food for the first six months of an infant's life.** No formula preparation comes close to breast milk in meeting the nutritional needs of infants and yet over the past century, the formula industry has reversed feeding trends from primarily breastfeeding to formula feeding through pervasive marketing strategies targeting hospitals, health providers, and the general public." --Kaplan, D.L. and Graff, K.M., Journal of Urban Health: Bulletin of the New York Academy of Medicine, 2008

4. "Breast milk is a 'live' food that contains living cells, hormones, active enzymes, antibodies and at least 400 other unique components. It is a dynamic substance, the composition changes from the beginning to the end of the feed according to the age and needs of the baby. Because it also provides active immunity, every time a baby breastfeeds it receives protection from disease. Compared to this miraculous substance, **the artificial milk sold as infant formula is little more than junk food**. It is the only manufactured food that

humans are encouraged to consume exclusively for a period of months, even though we know that no human body can be expected to stay healthy and thrive on a steady diet of processed food." --Thomas, P. "Suck on This", The Ecologist, 2006

Supply and Demand

Take a look at the example from CNN News of a mother who supplied milk for nine infants in a time of dire emergency (Officer Breastfeeds Quake Orphans) [. Surely, if she could sustain a baseball team of infants, *masha'Allah*, the average woman can supply one, *in sha' Allah*.

The point is that our bodies are amazingly designed by the best Creator to provide all the nourishment our babies need. It is a delicate balance between mother and baby; demand stimulating supply.

Unfortunately, this natural balance is upset when we introduce something "*man*" has claimed equivalent or better than that which *Allah* has provided. "*Just one bottle*" really can make a detrimental difference, especially in the very early days.

Return to *Instinct*

Trust *Allah* and the natural provisions He has given you for your baby. Abandon modern cultural myths and don't buy into the multibillion dollar baby food industry. Realize that the baby really should not be given any supplements for about the first six months of life. This means no water, no juice, no baby cereal, no baby food, no colic teas, no infant formula, etc. Nursing at the mother's breast is all the baby wants or needs in terms of nutrition and comfort.

On the Saudi Life Motherhood column I posted an article about Relearning the Natural Way of Infant Feeding.

Relearning the Natural Way of Infant Feeding

NURSING a newborn can be challenging at first, especially for a first-time mother. But surely all *Muslims* know that the infant has this right over us for the first two years of life [*Qur'an*: 2:233, 31:14, 65:6].

It's no surprise that modern science confirms what the *Qur'an* has told us for centuries. Evidence-based research has led the World Health Organization to advise:

"Exclusive breastfeeding is recommended up to 6 months of age, with continued breastfeeding along with appropriate complementary foods up to two years of age or beyond."

Sadly, many mothers in Saudi (and worldwide) fail to fulfill this responsibility and turn to artificial formulas instead. Sometimes it's a lack of understanding that babies need nothing but mother's milk for at least the first six months.

"Nothing" really does mean NOTHING: no formula supplements, no baby cereal or foods, no juice, no teas, not even water! Introducing even one bottle in the early days can disrupt the delicate balance of supply and demand, as well as interfere with the development of the nursing relationship. Exclusive breastfeeding provides ample nutrition and amount during those first six months.

The newborn's stomach is about the size of a shooter marble at birth. When you realize this, it's easy to see that the small amount of colostrum produced the first few days is just right for baby, *subhanAllah*. In fact, colostrum is sometimes called "liquid gold" for its yellow color and nutrient and antibody

Shooter Marble	=	Approximate stomach capacity of a newborn on Day 1
Ping Pong Ball	=	Approximate stomach capacity on Day 3
Extra-Large Chicken Egg	=	Approximate stomach capacity on Day 10
Softball	=	Approximate stomach capacity of an adult

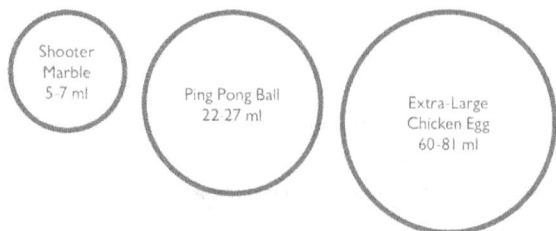

Shooter Marble
5-7 ml

Ping Pong Ball
22-27 ml

Extra-Large Chicken Egg
60-81 ml

Photo Credit: Ameda Belly Balls Card

rich elements. To deprive a baby of this specially-created-first-feed is especially dangerous. On top of that, substituting with infant formulas can lead to distention of the stomach as baby is often coaxed to drinking way more than he was designed to consume, *authubillah*.

Recently, I noted a short list of breast milk benefits in the article, <u>Husband's Role in Breastfeeding.</u> I also discussed the miraculous properties of this natural food that simply cannot be duplicated.

But what may be more important than the benefits of breastfeeding is the alarming truth that there are risks associated with formula feeding. Some of these risks have lifelong or even devastating effects.

Some Higher Risks of Formula Feeding as Compared to Breastfeeding [2]

- Allergy (food, breathing, and skin)
- Asthma
- Heart disease
- Death from diseases (such as diarrhea and lung infections)
- Obesity (40% more likely than breastfed children)
- Childhood cancers (including leukemia)
- Diabetes later in life
- Ear infection (50% more likely than breastfed infants)
- Infection from contaminated formula (many babies have died)

Additionally, most mothers don't realize that formula is not produced in a sterile environment. In fact, formula contamination recalls have occurred all over the world. A Google® search on "Tainted Baby Formula" finds over 800,000 results! Sadly, the tragic stories associated with contaminated formula could have been prevented if the mothers had chosen *Allah's* design for our babies' provisions, *authubillah*.

I don't believe that any mother would intentionally make a feeding choice that could pose danger to her child, especially when the solution lies freely and plainly within her own chest. Unless, of course, she truly felt the alternate feeding method were safe and possibly offered some benefit to her and/or her infant. In fact, I'm quite sure that every mother makes the best decision they can with the knowledge and information they have at the time.

The goal here is not to condemn mothers who have chosen to formula feed; I trust that those mothers have indeed made the choice they felt best for them at the time. However, my focus is to reach those mothers who have not yet decided and to provide support for the natural plan for infant feeding.

Although the decision not to nurse is difficult to reverse, it is not impossible. Relactation takes much more determination, patience, and perseverance than starting with breastfeeding right off, but it can be done, *in sha' Allah*.

As with most things in life, education is key. I suggest all mothers know how to get in touch with breastfeeding counselors and support groups in their area. As a breastfeeding counselor myself, I welcome questions and am happy to provide support.

The goal is to reach one mother, one baby, one drop of milk at a time. In fact, I'd love to hear from other women who would be willing to train as breastfeeding counselors as well.

The Messenger of Allah (*sallallahu `alayhi wa sallam*) said, **"Whoever relieves his brother of a hardship from the hardships of this world, Allah shall relieve him of a hardship from the hardships of the Day of Judgment. And whoever makes things easy for a person in difficulty, Allah will ease for him in this world and the Next. And whoever conceals (the faults of) a Muslim, Allah will conceal him in this world and the Next. Allah is forever aiding a slave so long as he is in the aid of his brother."** [Sahih Muslim, al-Tirmidhi, Ibn Majah and others]

Fortunately, all mothers can share and get support from *La Leche League*. This is a phenomenal mother-to-mother breastfeeding support group, which includes trained breastfeeding leaders in our own communities. If you cannot find a leader in your area, you can still join a virtual group and benefit from the exchange between mothers and counselors that support each other in breastfeeding, insha'Allah.

May Allah guide our sisters to the best for themselves and their babies.

Breastfeeding Benefits Mother

With that in mind, it's important that mother's realize the massive benefits to breastfeeding. First of all, as noted before, the action of stimulating the nipple serves to contract the uterus in the first days after birth. These contractions are a built in safety net between mother and baby that serves to expel the placenta (without the need for drugs or injections) immediately after birth and effectively shrink the uterus back down to its normal size. This is an important element in preventing harm from postpartum bleeding, as the shrinking of the organ serves to clamp down the open blood vessels of the placental site, which is a potential area for postpartum hemorrhage. Not only this but women who breastfeed for at least two years of their lives, whether continuously with one infant or cumulatively with many, have a 50% reduction in the risk of breast cancer later in life, *subhan'Allah*.

Breastfeeding Benefits Baby

Besides the important benefits to the mother, the baby also reaps incomparable benefits. The first "milk" is actually a thick, sticky, yellow substance called colostrum. This is often referred to as "liquid gold," as it is full of important antibodies for the baby that he/she cannot possibly gain from any other source, *subhan'Allah*. These antibodies come from the mother and are a direct reflection of the living environment of her particular baby. No manmade formula can duplicate this! This first "milk" is minimal in amount, leaving some women to feel they haven't "enough" and therefore making the mistake of starting the first supplemental feed.

Considering that the newborn's stomach is only about the size of a pea, it really cannot take more than the colostrum produced by the mother, without bloating the stomach. Once we offer formula and effectively distend the stomach, we have not only caused a potential nipple confusion, but also a baby who does not have a true sense of "fullness" and is predisposed to overeating, which may not be compatible with the mother's milk supply, and leaves the child with an increased risk of obesity throughout his/her life.

This first milk is also a laxative, which helps to clear out the baby's digestive system of the thick, tarry feces of the first few days of life. Of course, this does not even touch on the emotional blessings of bonding at the breast, which is what the newborn's strongest instinct from the moment of birth onwards in the first days, weeks, and even months of life.

Below is an article from the Saudi Birth Story blog about more of the Infant Health Benefits from Natural Birth and Breastfeeding.

Infant Health Benefits from Natural Birth and Breastfeeding

Bismillah al-Rahman al-Rahim

An informative article about Probiotics (live bacteria which benefits human health) in breast milk appeared in Al Riyadh newspaper on June 4, 2010. The original article was published in Arabic. I found many points in the article to be rather interesting as well as confirming my beliefs in natural birth and breastfeeding, alhamdulelah.

My husband was kind enough to do a quick summary translation for us to read here. I hope you enjoy the article and welcome your story ideas as well. Now on to the English version of the story...Infant Health Benefits from Natural Birth and Breastfeeding...

The full title of the Arabic article is *Probiotic is a group of friendly bacteria which increases infant immunities.* The article was divided into three parts.

Part I – discusses pregnancy and natural delivery and lists seven reasons for cesarean [just to note, I don't completely agree with this list but this article isn't about that]:

1. Breech

2. Chronic illness (mother) which would deteriorate in labor

3. Mother has vaginal infection

4. Twin birth

5. Many previous cesarean deliveries

6. Fetal distress

7. Large baby

Research shows that infants born by cesarean are more likely to be ill or get infections.

Part II – discusses how natural birth promotes the growth of these helpful natural bacteria while they don't appear in cesarean born infants for six months or more!

Breastfeeding also promotes the growth of this bacteria called Lactobacillus [which is also present in the vagina, thus explaining why they are present in only naturally born infants, subhan'Allah] and Bifidio bacteria which are called Probiotic.

Breast milk provides antibiotics, which land in the baby's stomach, an important part of his immunity.

Because of these reasons, an infant born by cesarean is in even greater need of breast milk.

Part III – discusses friendly bacteria in the breastfed babies, explains the Probiotic bacteria and the two most important types, and the history of the discovery of these bacteria.

Benefits of Probiotics:

1. Eases digestion of lactose

2. Prevents cancer

3. Decreases cholesterol

4. Prevents infection

5. Improves effectiveness of ulcer medications

6. Reduces infant's instances of allergies in the colon

7. Improves effectiveness of nervous colon medications

Breastfed infants get the Probiotic benefits via breast milk and if not breast-fed for any reason, it should be added to his diet.

Mothers should continue consultancy with the pediatric doctor during the first year of the child's life to assess development (weight, head circumference, teeth, mobility, etc.).

Breastfeeding Tips

Below are some tips to breastfeeding that I have found particular helpful. Keeping in mind that most women are able to successfully feed their baby may be of the most important. However, if you've had breast surgery, breast cancer, or suspect a glandular tissue problem (usually denoted by severely asymmetrical breasts), then be sure to have your breastfeeding success and baby assessed professionally.

1. The baby "breastfeeds," not "nipple feeds." This means that the baby's mouth should take a good portion of the areola, dark circle around the nipple, into the mouth, and not just the nipple itself.

2. Bring the baby to the breast (not the breast to the baby) when his/her mouth is wide open to get a good latch, as described above.

3. Holding the newborn baby "tummy-to-tummy" with mother will ensure that he/she is facing the breast and does not have to turn the head on weak neck muscles to nurse.

4. Mother must completely relax while nursing in order to experience an effective "let down" of milk. If mother is tense or nervous she and baby will likely be frustrated breastfeeding. Try employing the same relaxation that was practiced for labor while nursing: close your eyes, relax your forehead, jaw, and tongue in your mouth, ensure your shoulders are not hunched over or tense, etc.

5. Realize that crying is a late sign of newborn hunger. Once your baby reaches this level of need, it's difficult to calm him/her down

for a successful feed. Watch for cues and nurse your baby long before he/she cries. This includes "rooting," which means tilting his/her head with an open mouth in search of the breast, sucking on his/her fists, etc.

Husband's Role in Breastfeeding

Having the support of loved ones can really make or break a new mother's confidence and determination to breastfeed. Below is an article from the Saudi Life Motherhood column about the Husbands Role in Breastfeeding. Interestingly, this article has more hits than any other on the entire Motherhood column!

Husbands Role in Breastfeeding

ALLAH (*SWT*) perfectly created women's bodies to feed and nurture babies right from birth. This free-flowing provision is all our babies need for the best start in life. In fact, it's all they need for the first six to nine months and continues to be their main nutrient source well into the first year as they transition to grown-up foods.

Beside the mother and baby, no one has more interest in the feeding choice of the infant than the father. He will most directly be affected by the benefits of breastfeeding (or conversely the increased risks of formula feeding).

Short List of Breast Milk Benefits

1. Free infant feedings
2. Healthier baby and mother
3. Less illness results in less medical costs
4. Milder diaper odor
5. Always ready, perfectly mixed and warmed

6. No bottles to purchase, prepare or wash

7. Ease of travel

Infant Formula Simply Cannot Compare

Actually, breast milk supplies more than nutrition as it reacts to the mother's environment and provides antibodies specific to her baby's exposure to bacteria and illness. The components of breast milk constantly change to meet the growth and health protection needs of the individual baby and no two feeds are exactly alike. It is certain that no manmade formula can truly duplicate this perfect, constantly-adapting food for our babies.

Additionally, there are many health benefits for the mother who breast-feeds. Frankly, breastfeeding serves many other purposes besides feeding, but rather than get into all the research or a lengthy comparison of breastfeeding versus formula, I'd like to look at what has influenced our feeding choices and provide some insight as to why the husband's support is so important to success for mothers who would like to go the natural route.

The Cultural Shift to Formula Feeding

It wasn't until the last century that other feeding options even existed. The advent of infant formulas and artificial nipples was a medical response for the rare babies whose mothers truly couldn't nurse.

However, infant formula has grown into a billion-dollar industry. Along with that industry came mass media advertising as women were given the "freedom" to leave their babies in the care of others while they pursued work or other opportunities "more important" than breastfeeding. Many women began choosing to bottle-feed or at least supplement breastfeeding with formula feeding in higher numbers. As our cultures changed so did our perception of breastfeeding.

"Bottle-feeding becomes a status symbol; breast-feeding, a vulgar tradition." [From a report on Infant Formula in Developing Countries*].*

With this cultural shift we began to interfere with the natural balance of supply and demand between the needs of the growing infant and the mother's milk production. Sadly, many new mothers began giving up breastfeeding rather quickly and the tradition of passing down the skills of breastfeeding from mother to daughter has been replaced by generation after generation of formula feeding instead.

There is plenty of research that confirms that for the majority of healthy women, breastfeeding is truly the best option for her and her baby, *subhan'Allah*. However, it's not always easy and the first weeks are the most difficult, particularly if the birth of the baby was medicalized in any way or traumatic. This is another reason I strongly advocate for natural, non-medicated birth. For more read my article, *Natural Birth Increases Breastfeeding Success*.

Husband's Support is Key to Breastfeeding Success

Regardless of the birth experience, mothers who are committed to breastfeeding will have more success if they have their husband's support. As you can imagine, it's very difficult to breastfeed if the husband undermines her desires to do so. In such a situation the mother will always be torn between what she feels is right for her baby and what her husband wants her to do. Either way she will struggle with her decision and will have difficulty feeling at ease.

Thinking about this, I am reminded of my own husband, who is very pro-breastfeeding. Just a few days ago, as I was nursing our daughter, he reacted negatively towards some breast milk that had leaked onto my tee shirt. To him this "bodily fluid" is terrific, so long as it is going into the baby's tummy, but the minute it spills elsewhere he reacts with noted disgust.

Of course, as a very experienced breastfeeding mother, this didn't disturb me much. However, I thought of a new bride who may be met with this type of reaction. It really saddened me to think of how it may affect her self-confidence and overall body image, as she so desperately wants to please and be desirable to her husband. Especially if this type of exchange were to take place while she's struggling to get the hang of breastfeeding and is overly emotional from having just given birth. I can empathize and understand just how demeaning it would be to feel she does not have her husband's support at this critical time!

On the other hand, if she feels loved, well supported and appreciated by her husband for the commitment she is making for their baby, she will have more determination to continue. With his encouragement, she will find the strength to work through any difficulty she may experience getting settled into a breastfeeding routine, *in sha' Allah*.

The best part is that it really does get easier with experience. Before long she and her baby will be breastfeeding pros, *in sha'Allah*! Watch next week for more keys to breastfeeding success, *in sha' Allah*.

More than Breastfeeding

Being a mother is more than just breastfeeding. It's offering comfort and care to the dependent person entrusted in your care. Some mothers are determined to get their newborn on their schedule from day one. Personally, I feel that allowing the baby to set the pace and feed on demand is more conducive to healthy growth and development. It also provides the growing child a sense of security as he/she learns to trust the world around him/her.

I also don't believe that you can "spoil" a newborn. Until the baby learns the relationship between cause and effect, they truly are in need when they cry out. Don't hesitate to pick up your newborn, cuddle, nurse, and comfort him/her. He/she truly needs your time and attention and is counting on your to meet those needs. I have found that mother's who feel it's best to let their children "cry it out" end up with really clingy and demanding toddlers who grow into young adults that experience difficulty with independence. By mercifully responding to your newborn's needs you instill confidence and trust that last a lifetime and safeguard your mercy from *Allah*.

Anas ibn Malik said, "A woman came to 'A'isha and 'A'isha gave her three dates. She gave each of her two children a date and kept one date for herself. The children ate the two dates and then looked at their mother. She took her date and split in it two and gave each child half of it. The Prophet, may Allah bless him and grant him peace, came and 'A'isha told him about it. He said, 'Are you surprised at that? Allah will show her mercy because of her mercy towards her child.'"

'A'isha said, "A bedouin came to the Prophet, may Allah bless him and grant him peace, and asked, "Do you kiss your children? We do not kiss them.' The Prophet, may Allah bless him and grant him peace, said, 'Can I put mercy in your hearts after Allah has removed it from them?'"

Abu Hurayra said, "The Messenger of Allah, may Allah bless him and grant him peace, kissed Hasan ibn 'Ali while al-Aqra' ibn Habis at-Tamimi was sitting with him. Al-Aqra' observed, 'I have ten children and I have never kissed any of them.' The Messenger of Allah, may Allah bless him and grant him peace, looked at him and said, 'Whoever does not show mercy will not be shown mercy.'"

Newborn Facts

Upon closing I want to leave you with some Interesting Facts About Newborns:

Interesting Facts About Newborns

SUBHAN'ALLAH, Allah (SWT), in his infinite wisdom created all mankind in stages. It is amazing to gaze into the eyes of a newborn and know that he was created from mere drops of fluid. Even more amazing is before the child was born, his provision was promised and his fixed time in this world was set.

On the authority of Abdullah bin Masud, who said : the messenger of Allah, and he is the truthful, the believed narrated to us : "Verily the creation of each one of you is brought together in his mother's belly for forty days in the form of seed, then he is a clot of blood for a like period, then a morsel of flesh for a like period, then there is sent to him the angel who blows the breath of life into him and who is commanded about four matters: to write down his means of livelihood, his life span, his actions, and whether happy or unhappy. By Allah, other than Whom there is no god, verily one of you behaves like the people of Paradise until there is but an arm's length between him and it, and that which has been written over takes him and so he behaves like the people of Hell-fire and thus he enters it; and one of you behaves like the people of Hell-fire until there is but an arm's length between him and it, and that which has been written over takes him and so he behaves like the people of Paradise and thus he enters it." [related by Bukhari and Muslim]

I remember people telling me, "Enjoy the newborn period; it passes so quickly." With our babies changing so rapidly, we often forget or miss these little-known facts of infancy:

1. There is a "soft spot" in their skull that does not become solid until around two years of age. This allows their head to mold when passing through the birth canal, thus allowing them to be born.

2. They are able to hear in the womb and they can recognize their parent's voices at birth. This is a good reminder to recite *Qur'an* for our babies in the womb as well.

3. The average length of the umbilical cord is about 50 cm. This is just long enough to nurse, even before the cord is cut. Delayed cord clamping and immediate nursing ensures early bonding and has health benefits for mother and baby.

4. When a newborn's cheek is brushed, they turn towards the touch, open their mouths, and try to latch on and suck.

5. Babies first few bowel movements are a sticky, tar-like substance called meconium. If they are exclusively nursed, it changes to a thin consistency and is yellowish in color after a few days.

6. Newborn babies can see, however they may not track or follow an object for a few months.

7. Their vision is limited to 20-30 cm. Just far enough to see mother's face while nursing in her arms. I love this, as it is such a sign of the importance of nursing and *Allah's* perfect plan.

8. Newborn babies don't have tears. Sure they cry, but they emit no visible tears from their eyes until they are several months old.

9. A baby typically is born with dark or gray eyes. It's not until a few months after birth that their true eye color can be determined (about the time their tears come in).

10. At first, babies cannot automatically coordinate breathing through their mouths. If their nose is plugged they must cry in order to take in air.

It is a great blessing and responsibility to watch and guard our babies as they grow and pass through the many stages of this life. The creation and growth of our child is one of the many miracles from *Allah* (SWT). What an honor it is to be witnesses of this miracle from the start, *alhamdulillah*.

May *Allah* bless you with an easy birth and healthy child who is pleasing to HIM and his/her parents.

CHAPTER 30

What to Expect in <u>AMANI Birth</u> Training-Part Five

The *Instinctive* Series focuses on trusting Allah's perfect design of our bodies to carry, birth, and feed our babies. We will discover the role of hormones in labor and how our emotions affect their flow. Along with this we will explore the influence our birth environment has on the process of labor.

When we become aware of our innate abilities to birth, we can begin to tune out negative messages and distractions in order to tune into the primitive instincts that guide us through labor. When we understand the importance of tuning into our bodies and turning to Allah we find that all of the intuitive instructions we need are already present for labor, birth, breastfeeding, and beyond.

The *Instinctive* series is compiled of four modules:

Module 1   The Role of Hormones in Pregnancy, Labor, and Birth

In this module we will explore the hormones that affect the mother's bodily functions during pregnancy, labor, and birth. We'll explore how hormones are affected by emotions and discuss the importance of emotional assessment and healing during pregnancy for a clear slate going into labor.

Module 2   Protecting Your Birth Environment

In this module we will discuss the importance of informed consent or refusal and weighing benefits and risks before making any decisions with regards to your pregnancy, labor, and birth care. We will explore where we put our trust during this important time of your life and assess ways to reduce risks for better outcomes, *insha'Allah*. We will also discuss considerations in case you don't make it to the birthplace in time.

Module 3   Intuition

In this module we will explore our inner voice, or intuition and the many distractions that may pose a barrier to trusting our intuition. We will discuss birth noises and reminders to always be thankful to *Allah, insha'Allah*. We will also explore deep inner feelings and focus on positive birthing experiences.

Module 4   Breastfeeding and Baby Care

In the final module we will discuss breastfeeding, newborn vaccinations and important points for preparing your post birth nest. We will explore normal newborn behavior and interesting facts, as well as several tips for breastfeeding, *insha'Allah*.

Final Points

Please check our website at www.amanibirth.com for information on AMANI Birth Childbirth Educators or Doulas in your area, or to become a Teacher or Doula yourself.

We welcome your birth stories at readerstories@amanibirth.com and would like to know how AMANI Birth has influenced your birth experience.

We also welcome your feedback and suggestions for improvement regarding this text or any of our materials or classes at feedback@amanibirth.com and hope you will forgive us for any shortcomings or errors in print. Your feedback will serve to assist us in making edits for future editions, *insha'Allah.*

It is a pleasure and an honor to be a part of your journey to parenthood and I pray that *Allah* make it easy for you and bless you with healthy children who are pleasing to HIM and their parents.

References:

Abouelfettoh, A., Ludington-Hoe, S., & Morgan, K. (2008). A Clinical Guideline for Implementation of Kangaroo Care With Premature Infants of 30 or More Weeks' Postmenstrual Age. *Lippincott, Williams, & Wilkins* (vol. 8, no. 3 - supplement: June 2008, pp. S3-S23). Retrieved from: http://www.nursingcenter.com/lnc/journalarticle?Article_ID=799983

Al Hajjar, A. (2010). Who's to blame? *Saudi Life Motherhood*. Retrieved from: http://saudibirthstory.blogspot.com/2010/11/whos-to-blame.html

Al Hajjar, A. (2011). After cesarean tips. *Saudi Life Motherhood*. Retrieved from: http://www.saudilife.net/motherhood/12289-after-cesarean-tips

Al Hajjar, A. (2011). Blood, pregnancy, and nutrition. *Saudi Life Motherhood*. Retrieved from: http://www.saudilife.net/motherhood/22145-blood-pregnancy-and-nutrition

Al Hajjar, A. (2011). Husbands at birth in Saudi. *Saudi Life Motherhood*. Retrieved from: http://www.saudilife.net/motherhood/16053-husbands-at-birth-in-saudi

Al Hajjar, A. (2011) Husband's role in breastfeeding. *Saudi Life Motherhood*. Retrieved from: http://www.saudilife.net/motherhood/13169-husbands-role-in-breastfeeding

Al Hajjar, A. (2011). Infant health benefits from natural birth and breastfeeding. *Saudi Birth Story*. Retrieved from: http://saudibirthstory.blogspot.com/2011/01/infant-health-benefits-from-natural.html#more http://saudibirthstory.blogspot.com/2011/01/infant-health-benefits-from-natural.html#more

Al Hajjar, A. (2011). Lifelong pregnancy exercise. *Saudi Life Motherhood*.

Retrieved from: http://www.saudilife.net/motherhood/10457-lifelong-pregnancy-exercise-for-women-and-men

Al Hajjar, A. (2011). Many mothers routinely "cut" at delivery. *Saudi Life Motherhood*. Retrieved from: http://www.saudilife.net/motherhood/23603-many-mothers-routinely-cut-at-delivery

Al Hajjar, A. (2011). Pregnancy primary care provider. *Saudi Life Motherhood*. Retrieved from: http://www.saudilife.net/motherhood/18143-pregnancy-primary-care-provider

Al Hajjar, A. (2011). Pregnancy sleep positions in the news. *Saudi Life Motherhood*. Retrieved from: http://www.saudilife.net/motherhood/14755-pregnancy-sleep-positions-in-the-news

Al Hajjar, A. (2011). Should we rearrange the pain? *Saudi Life Motherhood*. Retrieved from: http://www.saudilife.net/motherhood/6288-should-we-rearrange-the-pain

Al Hajjar, A. (2011). Waiting for labor. *Saudi Life Motherhood*. Retrieved from: http://www.saudilife.net/motherhood/8585-waiting-for-labor

Al Hajjar, A. (2011). What is a doula? *Saudi Life Motherhood*. Retrieved from: http://www.saudilife.net/motherhood/5569-what-is-a-doula

Al Hajjar, A. (2012). 12 epidural realities. *Saudi Life Motherhood*. Retrieved from: http://saudilife.net/motherhood/29734-12-epidural-realities

Al Hajjar, A. (2012). Take responsibility. *Saudi Life Parenting*. Retrieved from: http://www.saudilife.net/parenting/24346-take-responsiblity

Allain, A. & Kean, Y. (2010). *Protecting infant health: A health workers' guide to the International Code of Marketing of Breastmilk Subsitutes* (11th ed.). Penang, Malaysia: IFBAN Sdn Bhd.

Al Oadah, S. '...to wait out their postnatal bleeding for forty days.' *Islam Today*. Retrieved from: http://en.islamtoday.net/artshow-377-3321.htm

American Psychological Association. (2010). *Publication manual of the American Psychological Association*. Washington, DC: American Psychological Association.

Amnesty International. (2011). *Maternal health in the U.S.* Retrieved from: http://www.amnestyusa.org/our-work/campaigns/demand-dignity/maternal-health-is-a-human-right/maternal-health-in-the-us

Badgut.org. (2010). Babies and bacteria. *The Inside Tract® Newsletter* (issue 175, 2010, 2nd quarter). Retrieved from: http://www.badgut.org/information-centre/babies-and-bacteria-1.html

Balaskas, J. (1992). *Active birth: The new approach to giving birth naturally* (revised ed.). Boston, MA: The Harvard Common Press.

Batterjee, M. (2010). *A fading art: Understanding breastfeeding in the Middle East.* Saudi Arabia: CreateSpace Independent Publishing Platform.

Bradley, R. (2008). *Husband-coached childbirth* (5th ed.). New York, NY: Bantam Books.

Brewer, T. (1982). *Metabolic toxemia of late pregnancy: A disease of malnutrition.* USA: Academy Publications.

Buckley, S. (2009). *Gentle birth, gentle mothering.* Berkley, CA: Celestial Arts.

Davis, E. (2004). *Heart & hands: A midwife's guide to pregnancy & birth* (4th ed.). Berkley, CA: Celestial Arts.

Davis, E. & Pascali-Bonaro, D. (2010). *Orgasmic birth.* New York, NY: Rodale Inc.

Department of Reproductive Healthy & Research, World Health Organization. (1996). *Safe motherhood: Care in normal birth: A practical guide.* Geneva: WHO. Retrieved from: http://whqlibdoc.who.int/hq/1996/WHO_FRH_MSM_96.24.pdf

Dick-Read, G. (2009). *Childbirth without fear.* London, UK: Printer & Martin Ltd.

Dominguez-Bello, M., Costello, E., Contreras, M., Magris, M., Hidalgo, G., Fierer, N., & Knight, R. (2010). Delivery mode shapes the acquisition and structure of the initial microbiota across multiple body habitats in newborns. *Proceedings of the National Academy of Sciences of the United States of America* (June 29, 2010, vol. 107(26), pp. 11971-11975). PMCID: PMC2900693. doi: 10.1073/pnas.1002601107

Epstein, A. (2008). *The business of being born* (documentary film). USA: Ricki Lake

Farlex, Inc. (2011). *The Free Dictionary*. Huntingdon Valley, PA: Farlex, Inc.

Flynn, A., Kelly, J., Hollins, G., & Lynch, P. (1978). Ambulation in labour. *British Medical Journal* (vol. 2, pp. 591-593). Retrieved from: http://www.ncbi.nlm.nih.gov/pmc/articles/PMC1607519/pdf/brmedj00141-0011.pdf

Fraser, D. & Cooper, M. (Eds.). (1993). *Myles textbook for midwives* (14th ed.). New York, NY: Churchill Livingstone.

Frye, A. (2004). *Holistic midwifery: A comprehensive textbook for midwives in homebirth practice: Volum II: Care of the mother and baby from the onset of labor through the first hours after birth*. Portland, OR: Labrys Press.

Frye, A. (2010). *Holistic midwifery: A comprehensive textbook for midwives in homebirth practice: Volume I: Care during pregnancy*. Portland, OR: Labrys Press.

Gaskin, I. (2003). *Ina May's guide to childbirth*. NY: Bantam Dell.

Gaskin, I. (2002). *Spiritual midwifery* (4th ed.). Summertown, TN: Book Publishing Company.

Goer, H. (1999). *The thinking woman's guide to a better birth*. New York, NY: The Berkley Publishing Group.

Hartley, J. (2008). *Hospital slashes episiotomy rate*. Retrieved from: http://www.arabianbusiness.com/hospital-slashes-episiotomy-rate-42172.html

Hathaway, M., & Hathaway, J. (2009). Introduction to second stage labor. In *The Bradley Method® student workbook*. Sherman Oaks, CA: AAHCC.

INFACT Canada. (2006). *Risks of formula feeding* (2nd rev.). Canada: Infant Feeding Action Coalition

Inter-Islam Publishing Company. *The book of taharah/cleanliness* (based on one volume of 'Nur al Idaah,' Imaam Shurnbalali's Classical Fiqh Manual. Retrieved from: http://www.inter-islam.org/Actions/Tahara5.htm#5-1

International Baby Food Action Network (various website content). Retrieved from: http://www.ibfan.org/index.html

Islam's Women: Jewels of Islam (various website content). Retrieved from: http://www.islamswomen.com/index.php

Janssen, P., Saxell, L, Page, L, Klein, M., Liston, R., & Lee, S. (2009). Outcomes of planned home birth with registered midwife versus planned hospital birth with midwife or physician. *Canadian Medical Association Journal* (vol. 181 no. 6-7). doi: 10.1503/cmaj.081869

Johnson, R. & Taylor, W. (2010). *Skills for midwifery practice.* New York, NY: Churchill Livingston Elsevier.

Jones, J. (2013). *The Dr. Brewer pregnancy diet* (various website content). Retrieved from: http://www.drbrewerpregnancydiet.com/index.html

Kutty, A. (2007). When to Resume Prayer After Postpartum Bleeding. *On Islam.* Retrieved from: http://www.onislam.net/english/ask-the-scholar/acts-of-worship/purification/173490.html

Laher, S. (2008). Proof of giving adhan and iqama in new born babys ear. *Quibla.* Retrieved from: http://spa.qibla.com/issue_view.asp?HD=7&ID=13079&CATE=1

Lawrence, A., Lewis, L., Hofmeyr, GJ. Dowswell, T. & Styles, C. (2009). Maternal positions and mobility during first stage labour. *Cochrane Database of Systematic Reviews* (2009, issue 2, art. no.: CD003934). doi: 10.1002/14651858.CD003934.pub2.

Liljestrand, J. (2003). Episiotomy for vaginal birth. *The WHO Reproductive Health Library.* Geneva: World Helth Organization. Retrieved from: http://apps.who.int/rhl/pregnancy_childbirth/childbirth/2nd_stage/jlcom/en/index.html

Lim, R. (2001). *After the baby's birth: A complete guide for postpartum women.* Berkley, CA: Celestial Arts.

McCutcheon, S. (1996). *Natural childbirth the Bradley way* .New York, NY: Penguin Group.

Midwifery Today. (2013). *Midwifery Today* (various website content). Retrieved from: http://www.midwiferytoday.com/

Mission Islam. *The Rights of the New Born Baby in Islam*. Retrieved from: http://www.missionislam.com/family/rightsnewborn.htm

Mohrbacher, N. (2005). *The breastfeeding answer book* (pocket guide ed.). Schaumburg, IL: La Leche League International.

Mueller, K. J. (2009). Advancing the health and well-being of rural communities. *Policy & Practice* (October, 2009, pp. 10-12). Retrieved from: http://www.aphsa.org/Publications/Doc/PP/1009PART1.pdf

Oxorn, H. (1986). *Oxorn-Foote human labor & birth* (5th ed.). New York, NY: McGraw Hill Health Professions Division.

Polachek, I., Harari, L., Baum, M., & Strous, R. (2012). Postpartum post-traumatice stress disorder symptoms: The uninvited birth companion. *The Israel Medical Association Journal*. (vol. 14, pp. 347-352). Retrieved from: http://www.ima.org.il/FilesUpload/IMAJ/0/38/19484.pdf

Riminton, H. (2008). Officer breast-feeds quake orphans. *CNN World*. Retrieved from: http://articles.cnn.com/2008-05-22/world/china.breastfeed_1_feed-babies-breast-feeds-breast-milk?_s=PM:WORLD

Simkin, P. & Ancheta, R. (2005). *The labor progress handbook* (second ed.). Oxford, UK: Blackwell Publishing.

US Food and Drug Administration. (2008). *Avoid Fetal "Keepsake" Images, Heartbeat Monitors*. Retrieved from: http://www.fda.gov/forconsumers/consumerupdates/ucm095508.htm

Varney, H., Kriebs, J., & Gegor, C. (2004). *Varney's midwifery* (4th ed.). Boston, MA: Jones and Bartlett Publishers.

Vaulted Treasures. (2007). Francois Mauriceau (1637-1709). *Historical collections at the Claude Moore Health Sciences Library*. Charlottesville, VA: University of Virginia

Velasquez, M. *Infant Formula in Developing Countries*. Retrieved from: http://wps.prenhall.com/hss_velasquez_busethics_6/38/9873/2527720.cw/index.html

Wagner, M. (2001). Fish can't see water: The need to humanize birth. *International Journal of Gynecology & Obstetrics*. (Vols. 75,

Supplement 1, pp. S25-37). Retrieved from: http://www.pbh.gov.br/smsa/bhpelopartonormal/estudos_cientificos/arquivos/fish_cant_see_water_the_need_to_humanize_birth.pdf or https://www.birthinternational.com/articles/birth/18-fish-cant-see-water

Wagner, M. (2008). *Born in the USA: How a broken maternity system must be fixed to put women and children first.* Los Angeles, CA: University of California Press

Wikipedia. (2011). *List of countries by infant mortality rate.* Retrieved from: http://en.wikipedia.org/wiki/List_of_countries_by_infant_mortality_rate

World Alliance for Breastfeeding Action (various website content). Retrieved from: http://www.waba.org.my/

World Health Organization. *Breastfeeding.* Retrieved from: http://www.who.int/topics/breastfeeding/en/

Arabic reference: http://www.saaid.net/female/m96.htm

www.ingramcontent.com/pod-product-compliance
Lightning Source LLC
Chambersburg PA
CBHW062202270326
41930CB00009B/1624